Advance Praise for *Life under Pressure*

"This truly unique and in-depth study of the complexity of suicide highlights the importance of sociological methods. The authors have collected and collated countless hours of interviews and material to respectfully share the painful story of one community's extraordinary experience of multiple suicides over many years. With their efforts and words, suicide prevention seems possible."

—**Jill Harkavy-Friedman**, PhD, SVP of Research,
American Foundation for Suicide Prevention

"*Life under Pressure* provides a vital intervention in the discussion of youth suicide prevention. The story of Poplar Grove tells us that the roots of suicide are social, which means that the solutions must be, too. From empowering schools to be sites of systemic care, to asserting the need for young people to be included in discussions about loss and prevention, to highlighting the protective factor of shared grief, Anna Mueller and Seth Abrutyn provide a road map to a more hopeful future where the mental health of young people is supported not only individually but by the institutions and communities in which they live."

—**C.J. Pascoe**, Associate Professor of Sociology,
University of Oregon and author of *Nice Is Not Enough:
Inequality and the Limits of Kindness at American High*

Life under Pressure

The Social Roots of Youth Suicide and What to Do about Them

ANNA S. MUELLER

AND

SETH ABRUTYN

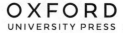

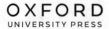

Oxford University Press is a department of the University of Oxford. It furthers
the University's objective of excellence in research, scholarship, and education
by publishing worldwide. Oxford is a registered trade mark of Oxford University
Press in the UK and certain other countries.

Published in the United States of America by Oxford University Press
198 Madison Avenue, New York, NY 10016, United States of America.

CIP data is on file at the Library of Congress

ISBN 978–0–19–084784–5

DOI: 10.1093/oso/9780190847845.001.0001

Printed by Sheridan Books, Inc., United States of America

To Julio & Dani

To the kids of Poplar Grove

CONTENTS

ACKNOWLEDGMENTS

A research project like this would be impossible without the support of a lot of individuals, organizations, and the community of "Poplar Grove" itself. Most importantly, we thank the many individuals who spoke with us one-on-one and in focus groups. Sharing your experiences, feelings, and reflections was difficult to do in most cases and painful in others. And yet, we learned so much from what you all shared. We hope we have done justice to your stories and helped bring meaning and purpose to your experiences. We will do all we can to continue to make your contribution to science and suicide prevention meaningful.

We are also grateful to everyone who helped us navigate the community, provided space for us to meet and talk with community members, invited us to community events or to their homes, or organized community events where we were able to share our findings with the community, listen to feedback, and answer questions. While we cannot recognize you by name (to preserve confidentiality), please know that we are grateful for all the work you did to make this research possible.

We also had the amazing good fortune of having a local host, Anna's childhood friend C.K. C.K., you not only provided us a free place to stay (critical for our shoestring budget), but also provided wonderful emotional support, dog walks, delicious food, and fantastic conversation to help us unwind after long days of fieldwork. In all honesty, having the bonus of getting to see you while doing fieldwork that was often emotionally tough made all the difference.

Both of us have changed universities throughout the life of this project, and we would not have been able to do what we did without, first and foremost, the University of Memphis sociology department's social, intellectual, and financial support. As our first job after graduate school, our chair Martin Levin was constantly in our corner, while so many of our colleagues spent countless hours, whether they liked it or not, talking about research, qualitative methods, and suicide. In addition to Marty, we especially thank Wesley James, Zandria Robinson, and Kendra Murphy from the University of Memphis for helping to create this wonderful academic environment. We are particularly grateful to Zandria for allowing Anna to audit her graduate qualitative methods course and for helping us think through study design and research methods. We are also grateful to Eugene Raikhel, Anna's colleague at the University of Chicago, for introducing us to the rich anthropology of suicide and medical anthropology. It helped fill gaps in the sociology of suicide and make sense of some of what we observed in Poplar Grove.

Of course, most research is also supported by numerous graduate and undergraduate research assistants. Ours was no different. Our research assistants helped transcribe, de-identify, organize, and sometimes even analyze our data. We couldn't have written this book without your help. Thank you. We would particularly like to acknowledge the following: from the University of Memphis, Taylor Binnix, Tijuana Jefferson, Darla Still, Cynthia Stockton, Anna Talley, and Allen West; from the University of Chicago, Sanja Miklin, Katherine Ordoñez, and Melissa Osborne; and from Indiana University, Katie Beardall and Robert Gallagher. We particularly appreciate learning from Robert's dissertation research on how laws can help build supportive communities for gender and sexual minority youth in schools, which we draw on in the conclusion.

We have also been fortunate to have support beyond the walls of our respective institutions. Sociologists Nicole Deterding, Sarah Diefendorf, and Jennifer Silva provided important guidance with qualitative research methods and helped us think through methodological questions, ethical dilemmas, and analytic strategies. Sociologists Kimberly Huyser and Lindsey Richardson provided endless cheerleading and encouragement.

Psychologists Sarah Hope Lincoln and Lauren O'Reilly generously shared their expertise in suicide, self-harm, and psychopathology. We are grateful to you all.

The field research for this project was largely financed through start-up funds provided by our universities, initially and most critically with the University of Memphis, but also the University of Chicago, Indiana University, and the University of British Columbia. However, data analysis was funded by the American Foundation for Suicide Prevention (AFSP) under award number SRG-0-200-17 awarded to Anna S. Mueller (PI). We are grateful for the financial and intellectual support our universities and the AFSP.

There have been several folks who have read and commented on drafts of this manuscript. We are particularly grateful to Anna's friends and fellow suicide prevention experts Emily Fine and Nate Thompson, Anna's father Bill Mueller, and her mentors Rob Crosnoe and Chandra Muller for reading and commenting on the book in progress. Beyond commenting on the book, Chandra, you've always been a wonderful intellectual force in Anna's life, providing support, caution, critique, and astute analysis. Rob, you astound us with your fast, thorough, and insightful commentary. It is something special to have a PhD advisor (Chandra) and a mentor (Rob) one can count on more than a decade after graduation.

It is hard to figure out how to appropriately acknowledge and thank the marvelous Letta Page (https://pagesmithing.com), who painstakingly poured over every chapter of this book providing us with important edits and insightful comments and helping us hone honestly everything about the book. It would be easier to figure out how to acknowledge Letta if that was all she did. But she also became our most trusted confidant and the person with whom we were most vulnerable (with our ideas). She made writing this book possible and even joyful. Letta, we aren't sure we would have gotten here without you. Thank you for all you gave us, the words and beyond.

Research like this requires travel. It also requires hours of isolated analysis and conversation, and probably too much of our attention devoted to the project. To that end, our respective partners, Julio Postigo and Danielle

Abrutyn, you have a special place in our hearts and minds. You two were and are amazing. Julio, we are particularly grateful for lending your GIS skills to make the map that appears as Figure 1.1 in Chapter 1. Danielle, you spent many nights listening to us talk about our research and helping brainstorm ideas on countless aspects of our project. We also found emotional, mental, and intellectual support from our families: Joan and Dave, Bill and Pat, Dani and Phil, Betty and Paul, Diana and Jeff, Eric and Jane, Asa and Silas, and so many others.

If you or someone you love needs help, please seek help.
We offer the following resources as a starting point.

In the United States and Canada, you can call the National Suicide
Prevention Lifeline for free & confidential support 24/7: 988

Outside the United States and Canada, the following websites provide
information on accessing free & confidential support:
https://findahelpline.com/i/iasp
https://befrienders.org

THE MYSTERY OF SUICIDE CLUSTERS

"The Last 10 Days of My Life"

Day 1: This feels so unreal, I am completely torn about what I should do. I know how many people I would hurt and they're people I would never want to hurt in a million years. So I need to decide, do I save myself in efforts to make everyone else happy, leaving me to live a miserable life or ruin everyone else's life by taking my own. It is my life so technically I have the right to decide my fate and happiness. I know how I feel isn't anything that can be changed or healed: I'm not having a "bad day" or feeling sad for any reason. I just don't want to live, I see no future for myself.

My only doubt comes from the fact that I know how much I would hurt everyone. What if they become depressed, or even kill themselves, I would never know. I would never know how everyone turns out or what life would be like. What if I still do have a conscience after I die and I have to live eternally thinking about how bad I've hurt everyone, but will be too dead to do anything about it? If I knew what would happen to me afterwards I could have a much easier time making my decision. All my guilt comes from thinking about others. This is so selfish of me.

—ARIA, *teen, from her journal*

During her junior year at Poplar Grove High School, Aria found herself sliding into a worsening depression. She had what she described as the perfect life, including fabulous vacations, her dream car, and more importantly, a big loving family, close friends, and a boyfriend she adored, but daily life had become unbearable. Though she knew how badly her suicide would hurt everyone around her, Aria's psychological pain ultimately overwhelmed her. Aria ended her life 12 days after she started her journal, excerpted here with her parents' permission.

Suicide is almost invariably a shocking and painful event. Aria's death was no different. It left a profound mark on her family and her friends, who struggle years later to make sense of it all. *Why didn't she ask for help? Why did she die?* It also left a profound mark on her suburban community of Poplar Grove, USA. Aria's death by suicide was not an isolated event, but rather the latest in a tragic string of suicide losses. According to local community members, the enduring challenge of youth suicide started in the year 2000 with a high-profile cluster of suicide deaths and attempts among Poplar Grove High School students. Ever since, suicide has been a yearly problem.

A *suicide cluster* is the term for a disproportionately high rate of suicide over a delimited time period; usually, this means at least two deaths and one attempt, or three deaths. Suicide clusters are notoriously difficult to study, partially because they are rare and nearly impossible to predict. This book deals with suicide clusters in Poplar Grove, some that we observed firsthand and some that we learned about extensively from long-time residents.

Poplar Grove's collective story of suicide begins with a teenager named Alice. One afternoon, Alice tried to end her life. She went to a local landmark, a high bridge without any suicide prevention barriers, and jumped. It was broad daylight, and there were numerous bystanders. Their quick reaction, once she leapt, along with the mild weather and Alice's strong swimming abilities, undoubtedly saved her life. Even so, she was injured and immediately rushed to the hospital.

By all accounts, Alice was the ideal Poplar Grove teen: bright, outgoing, achievement-driven, and pretty in others' estimation. Her suicide attempt was shocking, and like all shocking events in tight-knit communities, it was much discussed. *Why would a girl who seemed to have it all, who showed few signs of struggle, try to end her life?* Alice shared in a newspaper interview that she basically withdrew from the community to prioritize her well-being in the months that followed. The noise died down, and her story might have been forgotten or relegated to an isolated, painful event. But about six months later, Alice's class- and teammate, Zoe, died by suicide. She used the same method and same bridge as Alice. Like Alice, Zoe lived up to Poplar Grove's most cherished values: she was successful academically, athletically, and socially, with lots of friends and a place on several high-status athletic teams. Her death by suicide stunned the entire community. Then only four months passed before Alice and Zoe's classmate Steven used a firearm to end his life in his home.

These incidents created a high level of cognitive dissonance for Poplar Grovians. Families moved to Poplar Grove for its promise of being the perfect place to raise children. Their vision of what that meant did not include their children being repeatedly exposed to the suicide deaths of peers. It did not mean living in a place where they had to wonder, why is this happening, and could this happen to my family? Counting suicide among the possible tragedies that could happen in Poplar Grove triggered a lot of intense emotions, and many people looked for something or someone to blame. Parents and teens were understandably desperate to know why it was happening and how to stop it all. The experience of losing three high schoolers to suicide in one year became what sociologists call a collective trauma,[1] permanently written in Poplar Grove's collective memory.[2] Easily recalled, even by people who did not directly live through it, because it mattered so much to who the community is today.

So far as we could tell through our fieldwork, this initial cluster was followed by a reprieve from suicide losses. However, about seven years after the initial youth suicide cluster, two well-admired boys died by suicide within three weeks of each other. Eight months after that, a popular girl named Kate, with strong social ties to the boys, took her life using the same method as Zoe and Alice. And less than a year after Kate's death, another larger cluster emerged: Charlotte and three of her close male friends died by suicide in a six-week period. From that point on, at least one Poplar Grove youth or young adult died by suicide every year. Some years, the community weathered multiple suicide deaths. Numerous kids attempted suicide. In the decade between 2005 and 2016, Poplar Grove High School, a school of just about 2,000 students, lost four adolescent girls to suicide (five if we count a girl who had recently transferred out of the school), as well as two middle school students and at least twelve recent graduates.

By any measure, this extremely high rate of suicide is out of sync with local and national rates. Table I.1 summarizes the suicide losses that we were able to confirm in Poplar Grove. It became hard to untangle where the clusters started and stopped as suicide deaths and attempts accumulated. Many of the later youth who died by suicide had ties to multiple earlier youth who had died by suicide—they shared neighborhoods or churches, they were classmates or went to school with the siblings of youth who had died. This was a uniquely adolescent problem. While the occasional adult in Poplar Grove or Poplar Grove's county dies by suicide, the adult suicide rate is not notably different from state or national averages.

Table I.1 SUMMARY OF YOUTH/YOUNG ADULT
SUICIDE DEATHS THAT IMPACTED POPLAR GROVE
HIGH SCHOOL STUDENTS

	Number of Suicide Deaths
2000	2
2001–2006	No Reliable Data
2007–2009	8
2010–2012	4
2013–2015	5
	19

Because of the lengthy story of suicide in Poplar Grove, understanding why Aria's psychological pain and hopelessness lead to her eventual death requires understanding a much longer and broader story. Her death cannot be understood in isolation. Her death was the latest trauma, the latest tragedy in a long, painful line of losses. It made everyone wonder,

What on earth is happening in this beautiful, idyllic community to render suicide clusters such a shockingly common event?

I.1 UNDERSTANDING SUICIDE CLUSTERS

One of the most frustrating things for communities like Poplar Grove is that so little is known about what causes suicide clusters to form and, in some cases, persist, and what strategies can stop them. As scientists working on this topic since 2012, we share their frustration. Scientific knowledge on the causes of suicide clusters can be summed up in just a few short lines: We know that youth, young men, and people with preexisting risk factors for suicide are uniquely vulnerable to dying by suicide as part of a suicide cluster.[3-8] We also know that certain kinds of places where it's easy to know who belongs to the place and who doesn't—like high schools—are more vulnerable to experiencing suicide clusters than other places.[4] And finally, we know that when a suicide receives a lot of high-profile, sensationalized media attention, it is more likely to be followed by additional suicide deaths, forming a suicide cluster,[9] though it's not really clear whether the media attention is actually the thing that causes the initial suicide to escalate into a suicide cluster or whether prominent media coverage is more likely to follow certain kinds of deaths, such as deaths that impact the community more.[10] What is Poplar Grove supposed to do with this meager knowledge? Stop media coverage? They did that around 2007, and yet their suicide losses continued to persist, retraumatizing the inhabitants of this otherwise lovely community.

It's not that suicide prevention scientists don't care about suicide clusters. The Centers for Disease Control and Prevention (CDC) has done what it can to help communities from Delaware to California recover from suicide clusters by deploying its Epidemiological Assistance (Epi-Aid) teams of disease detectives to impacted communities.[11] But all these teams have discovered is what we shared in the previous paragraph. Scant and not very helpful. Much of our knowledge about suicide clusters is not very helpful because good data are incredibly difficult to come by. We lack detailed, nationwide data about the prevalence of suicide clusters or risk factors for them, meaning we can't even figure out what kinds of schools or communities may be most vulnerable. Instead, scientists almost always have to go into communities one by one, *after* a suicide cluster has happened, looking for clues across communities that will help us understand sources of vulnerability and resilience. Unfortunately, scientists rarely stay long. The CDC tends to finish their studies in under a month, which is barely enough time to get to know a community and the folks who live there and to build the trust needed for honest conversations about a painful topic. Another data challenge when studying suicide, including suicide clusters, is that the people we most need to talk with—the youth who died by suicide—are not around to help us understand what happened.

Indeed, these data challenges and the frustrating lack of information for communities are what drew us to Poplar Grove. We wanted to do something different. First of all, as sociologists, we wanted to understand not only the individual stories of why youth died by suicide, but also why this place—why Poplar Grove—was home to such a surprisingly high rate of youth suicide and recurring suicide clusters. Sociologists recognize that some places feed our well-being, amplify our joy, and make tough times more bearable, while others do the exact opposite.[12-14] This approach is important. Parents in Poplar Grove, like so many parents around the United States, were in search of a community that would provide their children with the safest, happiest childhood possible . . . and yet that was not what they found. What signs do we need to teach parents to help them recognize what communities will help their kids thrive? That's a question we help answer with this book.

Second, we wanted to take the time—in the end, more than three years—unpacking the complexities of Poplar Grove's suicide clusters. We did not want to just reconfirm what is already known about suicide clusters, but to go deeper. Sociology has well-established scientific methods for unpacking problems like suicide clusters, though prior to our work few had tried. Applying our tool kit to understanding youth suicide clusters has an additional benefit: we can elaborate our understanding of how the external social world matters to youth suicide. These goals are important. While mental health professionals acknowledge that social relationships matter to psychological well-being—for example, experiencing abusive relationships is very damaging to youth and can increase their risk of suicide[15]—much less is known about how to build social contexts that protect youth from escalating to suicidal thoughts or attempts when things go wrong in their everyday lives. And yet this information is critically important to effective suicide prevention. How can we build neighborhoods, faith communities, and schools that feed kids' well-being, no matter the individual travails they may experience? How do we create space for kids to ask adults in their schools or communities for help when they need it, including for mental health challenges? While in some ways these questions may seem obviously important, the science of suicide is so often focused on the individual who is at risk that we neglect to think about how the social world exacerbates or ameliorates risk. And yet answering these questions would help parents, school staff, and mental health professionals be more effective at building worlds kids feel are worth living in. These critically important questions are things we take on in the chapters of this book.

We draw not only on sociology, but also on the clinical psychology of suicide.[16-19] Clinical psychology has produced important knowledge about the suicidal mind that is useful for our pursuit of understanding both youth suicide and the suicide clusters present in Poplar Grove. Suicide—or the deliberate act of injuring oneself with the intent to die and that injury resulting in the person's death[20]—results from a complex tangle of biological, social, and psychological factors that cause someone to experience intense psychological pain that they feel no hope of escaping.[16,18,19] According to leading suicide expert and clinical psychologist Dr. Rory O'Connor, it's important to understand that "suicide is more about ending the pain rather than wanting to die".[19 (p. 65)] We can think of suicide risk as most likely to occur when someone's psychological pain overwhelms their ability to cope, when they have little hope that things can change, and when the person cannot imagine ways other than suicide to resolve their pain.[16,19] These insights into individual suicidal minds are useful for our work to understand suicide clusters. They suggest that in order to understand the suicide clusters in Poplar Grove, we need to understand why a disproportionate number of youth in this community are experiencing psychological pain and why so many youth use suicide to escape that pain. A corollary question we also can imagine is, why don't youth seek help instead of suffering until it overwhelms them?

Resolving these issues is what drew us to Poplar Grove. This book is our attempt to make sense of the losses and use knowledge gained from this collective pain to identify new strategies to prevent suicide and make young lives feel worth living. We offer insights into the social roots of psychological pain and how they translate into risk for suicide, and why certain places weather disproportionate incidents of adolescent suicides and suicide clusters. To do this, we use rigorous scientific research methods that involved us spending a lot of time in Poplar Grove. For those who are curious, we offer a complete discussion of our methodology in the Appendix. But before we delve into the social roots of suicide in Poplar Grove, let's discuss some basic facts and address some common myths about suicide to ensure a full understanding of young life in Poplar Grove and appreciate the risk of suicide there.

1.2 FACTS ABOUT YOUTH SUICIDE

Suicide is considered a significant public health problem among US adolescents. In the United States, the youth suicide rate has increased significantly since 1999, and particularly since 2007,[21] the same year Poplar Grove saw a rise in suicides. Today, suicide is the second leading cause of death for youth ages 15 to 19 and the third for ages 10 to 14. Importantly, while youth suicide has been increasing in the United States, this is not universal phenomenon. While the United Kingdom, Australia, and Canada have all experienced rising rates of youth suicide since 2007, other high-income countries—like France and Germany—have not.[22]

Despite these concerning trends, it is important to remember that suicide remains a rare event. Specifically, the suicide rate is (at the time of this writing) about 18 per 100,000 for boys ages 15 to 19 and about 5 per 100,000 for girls.[21] In the average high school student body of 2,000, that would come out to roughly one or two youth suicides in a 10-year period. Thus, most US youth do reasonably well in terms of their mental health in adolescence, and many grow up without ever directly experiencing a loss due to suicide.

While suicide death is rare, having suicidal thoughts is a much more common experience in adolescence. The CDC reports that in 2015, about 23% of high school-aged girls and 12% of boys had seriously considered suicide in the 12 months preceding the survey.[23] A smaller group of kids escalates from suicidal thoughts to an actual attempt, but it still is not as rare as we would hope. About 12% of high school-aged girls and 6% of boys attempted suicide in the previous year. Importantly, suicidal thoughts and attempts impact kids across race and ethnic groups. This is not just a problem for White kids, or Asian kids, and so on. Across all ages and all race/ethnic groups, girls and women report higher rates of suicidal ideation and attempts than boys and men, yet they have lower rates of completed suicides. Some of this gender paradox may be explained by the differences in lethal means that men and women usually employ, with men more likely to use firearms, which have a higher probability of death than other methods.[24-26]

The majority of youth with suicidal thoughts do not escalate to making suicide plans or attempts, though suicidal thoughts are an indication of psychological pain and emotional distress that warrants support, care, and concern. When disclosed and taken seriously, a person's suicidal thoughts can be addressed in families, in clinical settings, and in other communities of care, such as friends, schools, healthcare, or faith communities. It's important to understand that just thinking about suicide does not mean that a person is going to die by suicide; but it does mean that psychological supports are needed and that professional help should be engaged.

1.3 MYTHS ABOUT SUICIDE

One of the challenges of working on youth suicide is that the field is rife with myths—myths that sometimes are problematic for generating an accurate and complete understanding of suicide and for implementing effective suicide prevention. To ensure that we are all on the same page as we begin our examination of the social roots of youth suicide, we address some of the most prominent and relevant myths directly.

First and foremost, *talking about suicide does not cause suicide; it prevents it.*[27] Research shows that addressing suicide is a critical way to start life-saving conversations; answering youth's questions about suicide and providing trainings regarding the warning signs of suicide does not trigger suicide contagion. These activities are safe and beneficial for youth. What is not safe is *role-modeling* suicide as a means to escape psychological pain. Role modeling can happen through media stories or through personal experiences with peers, and it can be dangerous if it communicates motives and methods—meaning, the when, why, where, and how someone would attempt or complete suicide.[28,29] This is not to say that talking about suicide is not painful, particularly when we are concerned about someone who means a great deal to us. Learning to do it in a helpful way, before a crisis happens, is important. We offer insights into how to do this in Chapter 7.

Second, *suicide is not necessarily caused by mental illness.*[19] Especially in the United States, we have a tendency to think that mental illness is fundamental to risk of suicide.[30] In reality, psychological pain combined with hopelessness is what's fundamental. Sometimes that pain is tied to or exacerbated by a mental illness, but not always. Some studies find that the majority of people who attempt or die by suicide had lived with a diagnosed mental illness, but others add that nearly half of people who die by suicide had *not* been diagnosed with mental illness at the time of their death. Not everyone has an equal opportunity to be diagnosed, and this may account for some suicide deaths with undiagnosed mental illnesses. Simply put, the story is more complicated—as complicated as human suffering.

To correct another myth, we should address the belief that *suicide rarely occurs without warning.* There are almost always warning signs. Unfortunately, our society is not very good at recognizing those warning signs and intervening. Talking about suicide is hard and often feels scary, but it is important to do. And there is a great deal of stigma attached to mental health struggles the United States. In our experience interviewing families who have lost children to suicide, most times when families discuss their child's suicide as a complete shock or something that came without warning, they were actually noticing their child's psychological pain and distress. They just couldn't imagine what that pain might mean, that their child was at risk of attempting or dying by suicide. For so many of us, suicide risk just doesn't cross our minds—even when we are face-to-face with a distressed person—in the way suicide prevention experts might wish it would. This underscores the importance of preparing ourselves ahead of time to talk about suicide and learning how to ask children direct, nonjudgmental questions about suicide, even if we think suicide isn't on the table. In Chapter 4, we go deeper into the cognitive bias we have against imagining the unthinkable, against imagining suicide, and how it stymies prevention efforts. And in Chapter 7, we offer guidance on how to develop these skills.

A fourth myth is about which kids experience suicide risk. *Suicide does not only happen to children with "problems."* We know that suicidal thoughts are rather common among 21st-century US youth. No matter how loving or kind, no family can guarantee their child won't experience suicidal thoughts. What we *can* do is build families and other relationships where it is safe to talk about anything. That way, we can offer support and help if and when suicide becomes a topic. Sharing suicidal thoughts does not mean someone is going to die by suicide. They are an indication that help is needed. The adults in children's lives must prepare to have effective, compassionate conversations about suicide and know how to help their children get help when needed. It is imperative that we dispel the myth, common among families as well as teachers, school counselors, and other adults in children's lives, that suicide only happens to *other* people, families, and communities. Suicidal ideation is common and often close at hand. When we attune and attend to it, we can intervene.

There are many more myths about suicide, but correcting these four are particularly critical to understanding the social roots of suicide and the analysis we offer in this book.[i]

1.4 ON LANGUAGE CHOICES

Talking about suicide—a stigmatized subject—can be difficult. In writing this book, we had to make several choices with regard to language. In the suicide prevention world, we generally do not use the language "commit suicide" as it can be deeply offensive to some survivors of suicide loss, though others appreciate that it gives the person who died agency.[19] Many who do not like this language dislike it because it implies that the person who died by suicide "committed" a crime (and of course, suicide was once criminalized). Generally, the preferred, nonstigmatizing language is "died by suicide," "ended their life in suicide," or other similar sentiments. The key is to recognize that individuals who ended their own lives did have agency that we should take seriously, and that their act should not be seen as a crime, or the only defining thing about them.

While words that we—the authors—have written never use the language "commit suicide" in this book, some of the people we interviewed did use the phrase "commit suicide" when talking with us. This is likely because "commit suicide" is common in everyday conversations about suicide. We have decided not to change the word choices of those we spoke to, as their words are part of their experience. For those who feel pain upon reading the words "commit suicide," we are sorry if this choice harms you. Please be aware that it will at times appear in this book, but only when we are quoting from an interview, and these interviews are largely with impacted friends and family.

1.5 PLAN OF THE BOOK

The goal of this book is to lay bare the social roots of youth suicide. The heart of our argument is the simple assertion that *the social world youth inhabit matters to understanding and preventing adolescent suicide.* The social world includes physical and social space, as well as the historical, social, political, economic, and cultural contexts in which people's daily lives play out. The social world captures overlapping contexts, from our homes to our schools, neighborhoods, and communities, within which we form the relationships that make our lives joyous and worth living or stressful and onerous. In these spaces, we also learn values and absorb cultural meanings, develop aspirations, and experience disappointments and tragedies, large and small. Importantly, by turning our gaze to the external social world, we can identify the social roots of psychological pain for youth in a particular place, and we can examine why youth and parents sometimes find it hard to get help. We dig into how some kids arrive at suicide as an option for escaping unbearable psychological pain.

In Chapter 1, we introduce the reader to Poplar Grove. The goal is to establish the contradictions we identified in a place that, on the surface, seems so ideal. It has many of the elements Americans often lament as missing in American life—particularly an actual feel of community that we found genuine—people authentically looked out for each other and loved living there. In Chapter 2, we turn to the achievement culture that permeates kids' and families' lives. The directive is simple: be the best academically, athletically, and socially. It creates an ever-present and, for even the most stable and self-assured kids, sometimes unbearable pressure. We then explore how the high-pressure achievement culture combined with the strong sense of community connectedness contribute to youth's risk of suicide in Chapter 3.

Our focus shifts a bit as we move into the second half of the book. In Chapter 4, we ask why youth are not seeking help, especially when they know that it's available. The community is not lacking in resources that could help kids deal with the pressure, distress, and pain they feel. But supporting the idea that kids must achieve at all costs, we find a second cultural directive: "good" people aren't mentally ill (and psychological pain was taken as a sign of mental illness). Kids covered up their illness, their pain, and avoided help-seeking.

In turn, Chapter 5 explores how Poplar Grove High School responded to suicide losses. While we acknowledge that effective suicide postvention is difficult for schools—in part because the science and funding are lacking—we found systematic ways that Poplar Grove High School fell short of best practices. We use these missteps, and how they impacted kids' experiences of the day they found their friend or classmate or school-mate had died, to offer guidance and hope for a better future in terms of postvention in schools.

Having explored the school's response, we look in Chapter 6 at the ways Poplar Grovians memorialized youth during funerals and memorial services, identifying both the dangers of not establishing guidelines for how youth suicides are remembered and the positives that may help other communities and schools construct safer mourning rituals. The heart of the chapter focuses on the fact that mourning rituals are normal, healthy, connectivity-generating responses to community loss, but in a tight-knit community like Poplar Grove, they run the risk of exposing more youth than we might expect to intense grief and narratives that may make them vulnerable to suicidal thoughts or even attempts.

We close the book in Chapter 7 by drawing out explicit lessons we learned from our research in Poplar Grove—and introducing ways that the social roots of suicide can be addressed to improve prevention and promote well-being for kids. We also recognize that Poplar Grove is one, unique community, so we offer guidance on how communities that look different from Poplar Grove might use insights from this book. Through our intimate, comprehensive view of one community's tragedy, we hope to move our understanding of suicide in a new direction and expand options for supporting kids in an increasingly complex world. We have no illusions that there are simple solutions or quick fixes to a problem as complex as suicide. But we also see reason to hope that if communities work together, we can do better to support kids.

NOTE

i. For a more detailed discussion of the myths about suicide, we recommend Dr. Rory O'Connor's 2021 book *When It Is Darkest: Why People Die by Suicide and What We Can Do to Prevent It*.

REFERENCES

1. Abrutyn S. The Roots of Social Trauma: Collective, Cultural Pain and Its Consequences. *Society and Mental Health*. 2023;doi.org/10.1177/21568693231213.
2. Simko C. Forgetting to Remember: The Present Neglect and Future Prospects of Collective Memory in Sociological Theory. In: Abrutyn S, ed. *The Handbook of Contemporary Sociological Theory*. New York: Springer; 2016:457–475.
3. Brent DA, Kerr MM, Goldstein C, Bozigar J, Wartella M, Allan MJ. An Outbreak of Suicide and Suicidal Behavior in a High School. *American Academy of Child and Adolescent Psychiatry*. 1989;28(6):918–924.
4. Haw C, Hawton K, Niedzwiedz C, Platt S. Suicide Clusters: A Review of Risk Factors. *Suicide and Life-Threatening Behavior*. 2013;43(1):97–108.
5. Niedzwiedz C, Haw C, Hawton K, Platt S. The Definition and Epidemiology of Clusters of Suicidal Behavior: A Systematic Review. *Suicide and Life-Threatening Behavior*. 2014;44(5):569–581.
6. Pirkis J, Robinson J. Improving Our Understanding of Youth Suicide Clusters. *The Lancet Psychiatry*. 2014;1(June):5–6.
7. Robinson J, Pirkis J, O'Connor. RC. Suicide Clusters. In: O'Connor RC, Pirkis J, eds. *The International Handbook of Suicide Prevention, 2nd ed.* 2016:758–774.
8. Gould MS, Wallenstein S, Kleinman M, O'Carroll P, Mercy J. Suicide Clusters: An Examination of Age-Specific Effects. *American Journal of Public Health*. 1990;80:211–212.
9. Gould MS, Kleinman M, Lake AM, Forman J, Midle JB. Newspaper Coverage of Suicide and Initiation of Suicide Clusters in Teenagers in the USA, 1988–96: A Retrospective, Population-Based, Case-Control Study. *Lancet Psychiatry*. 2014;1(1):P34–43. doi: 10.1016/S2215-0366(14)70225-1.
10. Mueller AS. Does the Media Matter to Suicide?: Examining the Social Dynamics Surrounding Media Reporting on Suicide in a Suicide-Prone Community. *Social Science and Medicine*. 2017;180:152–159.
11. Fowler KA, Crosby AE, Parks SE, Ivey AZ, Silverman PR. Epidemiological Investigation of a Youth Suicide Cluster: Delaware 2012. *Delaware Medical Journal*. 2013;85(1):15.
12. Durkheim E. *Suicide: A Study in Sociology*. Glencoe, IL: Free Press; 1897 [1951].
13. Wray M, Colen C, Pescosolido BA. The Sociology of Suicide. *Annual Review of Sociology*. 2011;37:505–528.
14. Mueller AS, Abrutyn S, Pescosolido B, Diefendorf S. The Social Roots of Suicide: Theorizing How the External Social World Matters to Suicide and Suicide Prevention. *Frontiers in Psychology*. 2021;31:621569. doi: 10.3389/fpsyg.2021.621569.
15. Cha CB, Franz PJ, Guzmán EM, Glenn CR, Kleiman EM, Nock MK. Annual Research Review: Suicide Among Youth—Epidemiology, (Potential) Etiology, and Treatment. *Journal of Child Psychology and Psychiatry*. 2018;59(4):460–482.
16. Shneidman E. *The Suicidal Mind*. New York: Oxford University Press; 1996.
17. Joiner T. *Why People Die by Suicide*. Cambridge, MA: Harvard University Press; 2005.

18. Klonsky ED, May AM. The Three-Step Theory (3ST): A New Theory of Suicide Rooted in the "Ideation-to-Action" Framework. *International Journal of Cognitive Therapy*. 2015;8(2):114–129.

19. O'Connor R. *When It Is Darkest: Why People Die by Suicide and What We Can Do to Prevent It*. New York: Random House; 2021.

20. Cha CB, Nock MK. Suicidal and Nonsuicidal Self-Injurious Thoughts and Behaviors. In: Mash EJ, Barkley RA, eds. *Child Psychopathology, 3rd ed.* New York: The Guilford Press; 2014:317–342.

21. Federal Interagency Forum on Child and Family Statistics. America's Children: Key National Indicators of Well-Being, 2019. Washington, DC: U.S. Government Printing Office; 2019. https://www.childstats.gov/pdf/ac2019/ac_19.pdf

22. Padmanathan P, Bould H, Winstone L, Moran P, Gunnell D. Social Media Use, Economic Recession and Income Inequality in Relation to Trends in Youth Suicide in High-Income Countries: A Time Trends Analysis. *Journal of Affective Disorders*. 2020;275:58–65.

23. Kann L, McManus T, Harris WA, et al. Youth Risk Behavior Surveillance—United States, 2015. *MMWR Surveillance Summaries*. 2016;65(6):1–174.

24. Baca-Garcia E, Perez-Rodriguez MM, Mann JJ, Oquendo MA. Suicidal Behavior in Young Women. *Psychiatric Clinics of North America*. 2008;31:317–331.

25. Scrijvers D, Bollen J, Sabbe BGC. The Gender Paradox in Suicidal Behavior and Its Impact on the Suicidal Behavior. *Journal of Affective Disorders*. 2012;138:19–26.

26. Canetto SS, Sakinofsky I. The Gender Paradox in Suicide. *Suicide and Life-Threatening Behavior*. 1998;28(1):1–23.

27. Joiner T. *Myths About Suicide*. Cambridge, MA: Harvard University Press; 2010.

28. Mueller AS, Abrutyn S. Suicidal Disclosures Among Friends: Using Social Network Data to Understand Suicide Contagion. *Journal of Health and Social Behavior*. 2015;56(1):131–148.

29. Abrutyn S, Mueller AS, Osborne M. Rekeying Cultural Scripts for Youth Suicide: How Social Networks Facilitate Suicide Diffusion and Suicide Clusters Following Exposure to Suicide. *Society and Mental Health*. 2019;10(2):112–135. doi: 10.1177/2156869319834063.

30. Marsh I. *Suicide: Foucault, History and Truth*. Cambridge, MA: Cambridge University Press; 2010.

AN IDEAL PLACE

When we first arrived in Poplar Grove, searching for the source of its youth suicide problem, what we found was not what we expected. We expected to encounter a set of suburban neighborhoods smushed together that barely felt like a community. We imagined that youth and families might not know their neighbors, and that they might not experience the strong sense of the connectedness that often feeds positive mental and physical health. Instead, what we found was a small, tightly knit community with tons of pride, connectedness, and a sense of being in it together. Poplar Grove is, in many ways, an idyllic American town, delicately preserved and fiercely guarded by its denizens. Lovely houses dot tree-lined streets, jogging trails cut through well-maintained parks, and the community nestles between two scenic rivers. Better still, its residents care about each other, pull toward common goals, offer each other help, and share in each other's joys and sorrows. They told us right from the start that they were proud to call this town home—many having deliberately selected it as an ideal place to raise a family. This place is a real estate ad.

This idyllic community for all intents and purposes should be exactly the kind of community that protects its kids from suicide. So . . . how exactly had *this* town's much-lauded public high school, Poplar Grove High School (PGHS), come to be nicknamed, albeit in hushed tones, "Suicide High"? How had connectedness and membership in what nearly everyone described as a "highly desirable" community failed to protect its youth? Why had the community's best efforts and ample resources been unable to intervene effectively in this collective vulnerability?

In Poplar Grove, with time, we recognized the complexity of connectedness; we saw how it is equally possible to feel connected to *and* constrained by community values. The qualities of a community that make it inviting to outsiders and give insiders such pride can also be complicit in community vulnerability. Amid debates around the best ways to build healthy, happy communities and to design effective, community-level prevention strategies, we show that youth suicide risk and resilience are not only individual characteristics, but characteristics common to the community and its neighborhoods, schools, churches, and so on. Promoting connectedness may be regarded as an inherently *good* thing, but when it comes to public health, it's woefully insufficient.

Welcome to Poplar Grove.

1.1 COMFORT IN CONNECTION

"I don't think that we could find ourselves in a better place," enthused stay-at-home parent Victoria. Of moving to the town with her young child, she recalled, "I literally took my stroller out and was walking around, and anybody who had a baby stroller on their front porch, I knocked on the doors! Before you knew it, we had 17 moms walking four miles every day; kids would play on the driveway, at the end, for two hours every night." Twenty years later, the bonds remained strong: "[T]o this day—that group of women has changed a little bit over the years, but it's still a tight group of women [whose] kids are all the same age—we have gatherings almost every weekend." Her neighbors could be counted on as a "life support," she said, when her husband was traveling for work, offering to cook meals or give her a ride to the airport regardless of their own busy schedules. "Nobody ignores a request for support; somebody will always rearrange their commitments," she specified. To her, it was just part of what made life in "the Grove," as many residents called it, "pretty amazing."

Both authentically and purposefully, Poplar Grove embodies the mythos of the ideal American town.[1] We found Victoria's experience echoed by many community members who shared stories of friendly neighbors and readily available social support. Even those less enamored with small town life nonetheless confirmed the culture of connection. "Camaraderie is a strength of our community," Samantha, a young adult who grew up in Poplar Grove, shared. "Everybody [pulls] towards the same priorities." That comradery is rooted in dense and overlapping social networks. People in Poplar Grove actually know each other, giving the neighborhoods a real community feel. Marie, mom to several teens, emphasized that this wasn't the lip service of vague, unrealized offers of help, but the support of a community built through shared activities and mutual relationships: "[We all] socialize together, we have block parties. You know we *do* things together." And she was right: our fieldnotes were filled with parents showing up for each other's events and showering each other with practical and emotional support when tragedies struck. Quite explicitly, being engaged was the local expectation for a good neighbor in Poplar Grove.

The younger generation affirmed the support and connection they felt within their community. Victoria's teenaged daughter Shannon told us, "Our neighborhood is very intimate," and "Every time I walk down the street, I say hi to everybody I know, even the adults, just 'cause I've known them my entire life. It's a big network of support." And Isabel, a young adult, explained how growing up, she appreciated how "if I got hurt, I knew I could go to any street . . . and get what I needed. It didn't have to be my parents. I could just walk in [to any house], crying with a busted knee, and they would help . . . I love that sense of community that we feel."

Comments like these weren't entirely surprising, since many parents spoke about how they had deliberately cultivated a sort of collective watch over the neighborhood youth. Marie, the mom who talked about block parties, attributed her engaged relationships with her neighbors, in part, to getting to know each other's kids, and long-time resident Paula bragged warmly, "We had 200 kids in our neighborhood [when my kids were little], and I knew *every single one* of them." Poplar Grove's deeply interconnected social life allowed adults to keep track of and, to some extent, support each other's parenting: "The kids know that if I see a kid that's doing something that shouldn't be happening, I can say [something]." Sure, "a few parents" didn't like it if another adult scolded their child, Marie continued, but "most of them" were grateful you paid attention and stepped in.

Formal channels also kept the kid-related information flowing, despite apparent constraints. For instance, a religious leader named Linda told us her organization and the school system had signed "confidentiality things" because "church and state separation was an issue," yet revealed leaders at the organization and the school had a tacit agreement to break confidentiality if it was important to the well-being of the community, especially to protect a child within it. At every level, these lines of communication were intentional, and they created a dense webbing of community-held knowledge that crosscut neighborhoods and organizations.

1.2 CREATING A SMALL-TOWN FEEL

Much about Poplar Grove facilitates its intense sense of community. In practical terms, it is a small place with less than 40,000 residents. It takes less than 15 minutes to drive across the community. It's all but inevitable that, living here, you would quickly get to know a large portion of the population simply as you ran errands, stopping in at the Starbucks, the grocery store, or the popular, locally owned Grove Café.

As with many towns like it, Poplar Grove began as a stop on a railroad line that ran between two major urban areas, leading to it becoming a more natural environment for wealthier urbanites to either spend the weekend or live outside the big city. Not surprisingly, Poplar Grove's 13 small neighborhoods were carefully crafted to facilitate a community feel. There are beautiful outdoor spaces, including river beaches and boat launches and municipal parks featuring Frisbee golf, playgrounds, basketball, and community pools. Jim, a father, told us these shared spaces made it easier to get to know people and "feel grounded" in this "tight-knit community." As he put it, "[E]verybody knows everybody and we know all the kids, so you feel like there's [a] network, a safety net around you all the time. That is really wonderful." The value added by the green space "create[s] an environment that's very special," Paula mentioned as she underscored the town as a unified collective. "[N]o one owns the waterfront in my neighborhood . . . even if your [house is] sitting right there on the river, because the community owns it."

While neighborhoods served as intimate points of contact, small towns like Poplar Grove solidify connections through organizations that bridge neighborhoods, bringing members who may know of each other together. The fantastic community center and adjacent public library at the geographic heart of Poplar Grove had become its de facto Town Square (as the town, curiously, lacked an actual one). Young and old, everyone could gather in the community center, making use of its exercise facilities, large indoor pool, rental spaces, and a plethora of programming, including dancing, choir, service and volunteer opportunities, drama, musical theater, and more.

Additionally, the community's relatively liberal Protestant and Catholic churches (there are no mosques or synagogues here, though there are in nearby communities) stretch out a sacred canopy for the community, including the affiliated, unaffiliated, and disaffected. Though they provide religious experiences and proselytize, these churches intentionally work together to address shared community needs, using their resources to take up their religious missions in a broader way. Linda, the religious leader we met previously, felt her church served the town by not only taking "care of the people who are members of the church" but also staying "very invested in what goes on out in the community." That commitment, again, was characterized in terms of supporting Poplar Grove's youth as Linda shared an example: A young girl, she said, once walked from a community roughly eight miles away, arriving at Willow Creek Church at 3 a.m. The girl, Linda explained, "was feeling depressed and scared," and she remembered feeling safe at the church. "And that's *what we want*; we want to make it a safe place for *people*." Along with the other houses of worship in the town, Willow Creek offered its own community-focused programming. It hosted open events, like one on parenting in the age of social media, organized Meals on Wheels deliveries, and allowed groups like the National Alliance on Mental Illness (NAMI, a mental health advocacy group), Alcoholics Anonymous (AA), Narcotics Anonymous (NA), and visiting researchers to use their facilities. By serving residents beyond their congregants, the churches expand the safety net and perpetuate the feeling of social connectedness that permeates Poplar Grove.

In short, the organization of daily life in Poplar Grove amplified the sense of safety and support and connected families to each other, feeding its reputation as the ideal place to raise children. Indeed, children appeared to be the heart of Poplar Grove, its raison d'être. "We're here because our kids are here," the aforementioned Linda explained about the community, "or we're friends with you because our kids are friends." In this way, the world of Poplar Grove revolves around its children, and particularly its children's activities. This focus on children is not unique to Poplar Grove. Through his four decades inhaling life in small-town America, sociologist Robert Wuthnow found that most small towns have a "moral center" that, like the sun, draws in and orders the movement and attention of its orbital members.[2] For many towns, that moral center is as we found in Poplar Grove: focused on the kids. Having a strong shared moral center transforms mundane rituals, like dropping kids off at school or attending soccer practice, and spectacular events, like rival matchups and homecoming games, into opportunities to intensify the collective identity—the sense that we're in this together.[3] In turn, each member of the collective—each parent and each kid—integrates that collective identity into something more personal, into a sense that they are from Poplar Grove and that that matters.

For Poplar Grove, the Cardinals, Poplar Grove's sports league for kids, plays a huge role in that moral center of community life. Children's sports are taken very seriously—the local paper covers their wins and losses faithfully. "In this particular community," a dad named Harrison shared, "sports are big. They start very young. If somebody hadn't said anything about Cardinals—" With a knowing chuckle, Harrison's joke trailed off, silently warning *oh, they will.* He used the term "highly involved" to describe the norm around youth sports, while Linda reported simply, "Everybody is signed up from the time you can walk." The rhythm of life, at least for parents, revolved around sports: tryouts, early morning weekend practices, travel games, and wins and losses. More practically, all that involvement provided opportunities for information-sharing. Weekly games, for instance, became, in Linda's words, "a social event for the families."

Fewer Grovians specifically called out the second community function of youth sports: building well-rounded kids prepped for adult success. That is, participation was part of the Poplar Grove's communitywide, concerted cultivation of their kids.[4] Playing with the Cardinals can help kids achieve visibility and social status, prep them to play varsity sports in high school, and build college resumes. The league mattered independently of school, though it also seemed to supplement the centrality of the schools in fueling social connectedness. Indeed, all kinds of school events were surrounded by this strong sense of obligatory—though eager—participation. Local papers covered the raucous Friday night varsity games, as well as Poplar Grove High's shockingly professional theater and music shows, as evidenced by the stacks of clippings and scrapbooks we saw throughout our fieldwork highlighting local students' perpetual domination of state championships across athletics, arts, and academic extracurriculars.

What is interesting in all this talk of Poplar Grove as a community is that Poplar Grove is—according to the US census—just a legal collection of neighborhoods, a census-designated place. One could argue it's not even a community. Social constructions and collective identities, however, supersede government categories in everyday life. In Poplar Grove, we found an intense community in which residents cooperate to forge and project the image and feel of mythical small-town America. Its schools, churches, and neighborhood associations knit the population together, creating social ties that generate warmth and meaning for the community. This is precisely what makes for a cohesive community that captures members' attention and emotion: it's about putting the group's shared ethos, beliefs, and cherished practices at the center of social life. Young people were the reason families moved here and lived here, and they were the focus of the mundane and spectacular rituals of the collective. This affirmed community members' social ties and shored up the collective identity. However, collective identity is not just patterns of doing the same stuff. It also has a material base, a tangible something that acts as the foundation for insiders' pride and outsiders' exclusion.

1.3 THE POWER OF REPUTATION

It was clear from our conversations, and eventually observations, that Poplar Grove *did* feel like a warm and supportive community. What's more, it was clear that people were very proud of their community and protective of its reputation. At first, this strong affinity for Poplar Grove surprised us. Beyond the well-manicured lawns and beautiful houses that we initially encountered, we didn't see much to recommend Poplar Grove. Without a true town square or the visible accoutrements of a cohesive community, Poplar Grove feels, to the uninitiated, more like any old nameless suburban neighborhood than the small-town idyll its residents describe. You can drive through Poplar Grove, passing its strip malls, chain restaurants, big-box stores, and requisite Starbucks, without actually noticing you've traversed the community's boundaries. And if you don't pull off that main artery, you will miss the local cafés, beautiful central library, and other things that physically support the social connectedness in Poplar Grove. We also arrived ready to enjoy nature—anyone can pull up Google Maps and see that Poplar Grove is nestled between two rivers and bejeweled with green spaces—but we found ourselves stymied when it came to accessing these natural spaces. Beyond the one big public park, it was really difficult to find the green spaces in real life. It would prove a deliberate configuration.

Over time, we noted that the community spaces and natural splendor that Poplar Grovians warmly cited as critical to their sense of community truly were hidden gems. During our fieldwork, Poplar Grove's beaches were entirely absent from Google Maps (though that is changing), and the neighborhood parks and their swimming pools appeared only as unlabeled green spaces. We had been conducting fieldwork for years before we saw our first Poplar Grove neighborhood park with our own eyes. Exasperated, Anna decided to drive around to all the green blotches on Google Maps looking for these beloved community parks. By digging deep into neighborhoods, she realized there were gorgeous, three-acre parks behind people's houses, nearly invisible from the street. They had basketball courts, frisbee golf courses, ponds, playgrounds, and yes, swimming pools. No one chased her out when she walked past the "NO TRESPASSING" signs and took herself on a tour, but the whole scenario made Anna nervous enough to text Seth that she was "going in" and would reconnect when she successfully made it out. Though it seemed possible to drive into the park, the road looked rather like a driveway—and Anna certainly did not want to explain to a local why she was driving into their backyard if caught. Instead, Anna walked cautiously down the driveway/road, passing more unwelcoming signs into what seemed to be someone's personal backyard—and while no one stopped her, to a Texan like Anna, every step felt like a dare.

Suffice it to say, if you do not belong to Poplar Grove, you'll get the sense you do not belong *in* Poplar Grove. Its beloved community spaces are all but inaccessible to a random interloper. Recalling Paula, who earlier in the chapter gushed about how "no one owns the waterfront in my neighborhood," we realized the things she'd left unsaid: the beaches are open to the public *if* the person *belongs* to the community and has paid the associated dues. The signs on wrought iron fences read things like "Olde Poplar Grove Community Beach. Members Only. No Trespassing." Outsiders that we were, we never did set foot on one of those beaches. We have no doubt, however, that if we had asked a resident to invite us in, they would have done so with great welcome and hospitality. It is also clear that, despite the welcome we experienced, Poplar Grove's reputation—shared by insiders and outsiders alike—had been staked on a sense of exclusivity. Communities, like any organized group of people, produce goods that generate pride and contribute to the quality of life. Scarcer goods become more valuable and costly. Exclusivity, then, is rooted in giving members something others want but cannot necessarily have. Not surprisingly, exclusivity furthers community connectedness: the costs members incur to enjoy those goods are a sort of shared sunk cost, and the reputational prestige of membership hardens the boundaries for non-members.[5] Thus, the neighborhood feel, the dense webbing created by various community organizations, the centrality of sports and children, and the protected cultivation of natural space produced benefits worth fencing in.

1.3.1 Affluence

Exclusivity like this is expensive. It requires the capacity to prevent free riders and establish minimum contributions to the collective good required to access it. Building a respected reputation as a kid-centered, academically and athletically excellent place is a privilege not afforded to every community. Clearly, the sports, schools, safety, and locals-only natural spaces were deeply entwined with the community's affluence. Typically blunt teen Hadley found this aspect of the town's reputation obvious: "[W]e're waterfront property. We've *got* to have some money in this area, and it's a lot of money . . . this area is full of rich [people with] all these high-paying jobs . . . Poplar Grove is known for being a big-money area."

The beauty, the gorgeous homes and neighborhoods, the academically and athletically excellent schools, and the above-average socioeconomic status of the majority of its denizens all lend Poplar Grove its elite status as, in the parlance of real estate ads, a "highly desirable" community. The median home value of owner-occupied units in Poplar Grove is well above the county median and 20% above the median in the county's second-most expensive town. Median household income is also highest in Poplar Grove, as is the percentage of the population holding at least a bachelor's degree. Its poverty rate is less than 5%.

Comments like Hadley's were ubiquitous in our interviews with young people. "People have their, I guess, opinions of Poplar Grove," started teenager Krista, "like people I know from other communities are like, 'oh, Poplar Grove, it's, like, the rich area. Like, the affluent area.'" Carrie, a few years older than Krista and Hadley, recalled the same of her youth in Poplar Grove: "People definitely have this thought that [Poplar Grove is] all people with money and uppity and preppy and, like, valley girl-like; that they're goody two shoes and this and that." Now in her late 20s, Carrie avoids telling others where she grew up—she says she doesn't want the "stigma" of an elite childhood subtly laying claim to or putting an asterisk on her (truly impressive) achievements.

Our interviews with outsiders in nearby communities lent credence to these reputational suspicions. A professor remarked that "Poplar Grove is very uppity," while a focus group participant described Poplar Grove as being defined by "status and privilege," to the degree that they shared an anecdote about a close friend who moved to the community but ended up pulling their kid out of the schools because they were being bullied. They just didn't "fit in." The same respondent shared that, on his first day of work, he drove "a beat-up old pickup truck into a parking lot full of Mercedes" and thought, "I'm not in the right world here . . . I'm not going to fit in." Youth were just as aware of the common sense about *what* Poplar Grove was and *who* lived there. Ander, a recent PGHS graduate, said matter-of-factly that kids "look to what they have . . . because if you *have*, you're *better*." They compare, he said:

> "I have this, and you don't have this." It's very obvious. You see what the people drive. You see what the people wear . . . because you have people picking their kids up from school who live in Glen Rhoda and Vollentine [surrounding communities] and more impoverished areas.

Poplar Grove's reputation was, indeed, built from an acute sense of being different, of being better. Their sports teams were better organized and funded; they won more trophies; their school excelled more than others. But more importantly, they could *see* these differences in the physical space around themselves, like cars or clothes or houses. That nonresidents recognized the community distinctions, too, meant the boundaries and, therefore, exclusivity were maintained, in part, by wealth. The consequence was the construction of a more coherent collective identity shaped around common purpose and lifestyle. Samantha, who we met earlier, noted that the visible "poverty in the school systems around Poplar Grove" made her "appreciate . . . the lifestyle of [her] community." She felt she shared more with her fellow Grovians than with "people who are concerned about day-to-day money." Samantha preferred not "to use the word privilege" when describing Poplar Grove, as her quote here underscores the pride and comradery she felt community members could feel in a state and, perhaps, national reputation of collective academic and athletic achievement.

One thing we noticed in our conversations with locals about why they lived in Poplar Grove is that an overwhelming majority talked about kids, schools, family-oriented community, and safety. We also noticed that while affluence clearly facilitated access to the community (and all its resources), and possibly also even conferred some status and allure to being from Poplar Grove, affluence was rarely mentioned as a reason why people moved to Poplar Grove. One place where affluence was more explicitly discussed was during our conversations with young adults (like Ander, Carrie, and Krista earlier) who left Poplar Grove for college, where they were confronted by a diversity of people and experiences. In many ways, it had the effect of revealing just how central affluence was to the Poplar Grovian collective identity. Gwen, a young adult, shared the following reflection:

I feel like my opinions of Poplar Grove changed a lot versus when I was here in high school, and then when I moved away [to university]. Now I've only been there for a semester, and now I have, like, a completely different, like, view of how I, like, think of [Poplar Grove]. Like, when I was here in high school I couldn't wait to get out . . . And then when I got to [university] everybody was super friendly . . . but, also the area surrounding [my university], is—I feel like it's almost culture shock for me from here. It's a very fun town, a lot of the people there are immigrants, a lot of Hispanic people. My team went and did a community service thing at one of the elementary schools for, like, a fall festival kind of thing. And it was, like, weird to see how different it was there, than it is here and I was like,

"Wow, I'm really happy I grew up where I did." Because I don't know
what I would be doing if I grew up somewhere else, I guess.

Gwen's culture shock is the product of a clash between her expectations based on her own childhood in her hometown and the reality she
confronts upon leaving.[6] Gwen thought the world worked one way. She
took for granted all the unnoticed privileges of growing up in Poplar
Grove; she even felt some anger at the pressure of expectations that came
along with her privileged childhood address. But when she went away
and learned about how other kids grow up, suddenly being from Poplar
Grove felt different. She took it less for granted; she realized all she had by
growing up where she did. From the safety of young adulthood, she even
doubled down on the value of being from Poplar Grove. As she said, "I'm
really happy I grew up where I did." In Poplar Grove.

Though adults rarely cited the affluence as part of what made Poplar
Grove desirable, they were often aware of it. Most commonly, they
contrasted Poplar Grove's affluence with their childhood neighborhoods,
often highlighting how they were able to give their children so much more
than they had growing up by living in Poplar Grove. Jim, a parent we met
earlier, fumbled a bit when asked why he chose to call Poplar Grove home,
but landed on affluence as at least part of the draw: "Yeah, that's what kinda
brought us here . . . It's much more, I'm trying to think of the right word,
economically, it's a more, the families are, again, I'm trying to—*affluent*,
that's it. It's a much more *affluent* neighborhood than I grew up with." His
own ambivalence toward having to "keep up with Joneses" aside, Jim felt
the "kids seem to be all well-grounded here [because] they're in a nice, safe
area . . . there's plenty of things for them to do." Safety, linked to affluence,
is a key ancillary of that affluent reputation, a tangible form of social capital usually noted among the reasons people wanted to commit to the community and maintain its connectedness, and in so doing, its reputation.

Explicit references by Poplar Grovians to desirable community and
schools often implied affluence. But there was also another key distinction between this specific town and neighboring communities: its racial
homogeneity.

1.3.2 Racial Homogeneity

Let's set the stage with some demographic information. Poplar Grove as a community is about 90% White non-Hispanic, making it far more racially homogeneous than Poplar Grove's county or state (which has racial demographics similar to Texas, with about 60% non-Hispanic White residents, and sizeable minorities of Hispanic and African American residents).

Figure 1.1 presents a stylized map (meaning we have smoothed community and census tract boundaries to obscure the community's identity) that illustrates the homogeneity of Poplar Grove and the diversity of proximate communities. The darker the shading, the higher the percentage of White

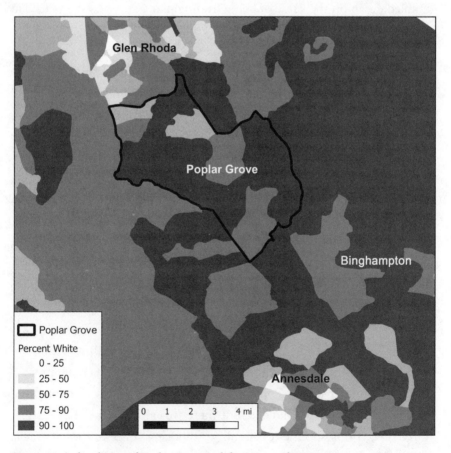

Figure 1.1 Stylized Map of Poplar Grove and the Surrounding Area.

residents in a particular census tract. The map makes it clear that while Poplar Grove is more than 90% White in most of its census tracts, it is *not* racially isolated. People of color live in close proximity to Poplar Grove, specifically in the small town of Glen Rhoda on Poplar Grove's northern border and in the slightly larger Annesdale to the South. Glen Rhoda is about 10 minutes away from Poplar Grove High, while Annesdale is about 15 to 20 minutes away. The small pockets of racial diversity on Poplar Grove's northern edge (bordering Glen Rhoda) coincide with the location of the community's only subsidized housing for low-income individuals. This housing is restricted to senior citizens.

Despite the dramatic demographic differences between Poplar Grove and surrounding communities, this aspect of life in the Grove rarely came up in our conversations with Poplar Grovians, young and old. The few that did mention it understood the White homogeneity as mattering, at least for some Poplar Grovians. In an early focus group, for instance, one parent said Poplar Grove "is a tough place" for children of color "to grow up . . . [not] many people like [them]" (quickly, she shifted to talking about other types of "differentness"). In another conversation, a parent contrasted the experiences of their adopted Latina daughter and bio-logical White son in the town: "She's not Black, she's not White, so what happens? That's an identity issue right there that kind of needed to be dealt with, [while] my son [who is White] didn't have any of that." Setting aside the daughter's dilemma, this parent went on to refer to their son as "home-grown," looking like a "Poplar Grove kid," and a "good athlete"—a combination that "gave him his own thing." A combination, she implied, that made growing up there easier on him.

These small tidbits of racialized talk in Poplar Grove hint that Whiteness was part of being a Poplar Grovian, and that being different based on the color of one's skin in Poplar Grove was not easy. And while it is difficult to tease out the relative influence of race, affluence, school quality, or neighborhood safety in creating Poplar Grove's particular brand of de-sirability, we'd be remiss to not acknowledge this part of Poplar Grove's story.[7,8] Because racial homogeneity does matter, whether it is conscious or unconscious, the main story or not. What living in a homogeneous community does is amplify the importance of being a member of that community to community members. It intensifies community boundaries and the identification of in-group members—people like us—separating them more clearly from out-group members. While being surrounded by people like us facilitates the creation of wonderful social connectedness, it also amplifies the importance of conformity, of fitting in. Our purpose is not to accuse Poplar Grovians of racism—far from it. Rather, our purpose is to shine a light on a hidden downside of everyone having such an intensely reinforced social identity, of being surrounded by people who are just like them.

But before we move on to examine what is expected of the inhabitants of this beautiful, privileged, connected community, it is worth unpacking what Poplar Grovians readily admitted drew them to their chosen community—the incredible schools.

1.3.3 The Allure of Excellent Schools

As we noted previously, the adults that we met in Poplar Grove most often explicitly noted the unparalleled quality of Poplar Grove's schools as the explanation for why they moved there. Newlywed Isabel, who we met earlier, enthused, "I absolutely loved growing up here and that's why [my husband and I] want to move back—because it's great." When we asked why she'd decided to start her own family in Poplar Grove, her number-one reason for choosing Poplar Grove over their second option, her husband's similarly community-minded Iowa hometown, was the public schools. The public schools, Isabel underscored, "are really good, so that's hard to beat." Erica, a mother in one of our study's early focus groups, told us that she, too, had grown up in Poplar Grove. Though she eventually started her family in Annesdale, the schools there "were *really* going down[hill]," and she and her spouse decided it was "either put all of our kids in private schools or move back to Poplar Grove." They picked Poplar Grove. After all, this mom figured, "I grew up in Poplar Grove, and I turned out okay." We met scores of people who moved to (or back to) Poplar Grove on the basis of the school's reputation. Harrison recalled,

"Back in the mid-1990s," when he and his wife Cynthia were deciding where to set up home, "we were looking at data on school systems. And what we found was [that] . . . Poplar Grove had, at that point in time, the highest SAT scores in the county."

While Poplar Grove's schools may boast impressive test scores, there was also something intangible about the draw of Poplar Grove schools compared to other, neighboring town's schools. Sarah, a young mother that we met, sounded like many other parents when she tried to describe the intangible side of the draw to Poplar Grove schools: "People live in Poplar Grove because they want the best schools. They want the best for their children," she explained. Sarah had grown up and gone to school in Annesdale, but said bluntly, "I wasn't going to send my kid there. There wasn't anything *wrong* with it, but Poplar Grove . . . is *Poplar Grove*." The exclusivity implied by this reputation for scholastic excellence came through in her coda: "Everybody wants to get [into the Poplar Grove schools], because they think they're missing out if they're not in." This proximate outsider's long-term view of Poplar Grove, in other words, was that it provided *something extra* that was unavailable in nearby Annesdale. Good parents "want the best for their children," so good parents do what it takes to get their kids into those good Poplar Grove schools.

While Poplar Grove's reputation for excellent public schools was clear and broadly shared, we, as outsiders, were not completely convinced that the education provided by the schools in Poplar Grove was really that different from Annesdale or other surrounding communities. Still, we asked ourselves—maybe Poplar Grove really is *the* place to get your kids an excellent education in this county. So let's take a moment to really dig into the school data. Not necessarily as a parent searching for a school for their child would, but as a sociologist of education—like Anna—would.

1.3.4 Reality Check: Evaluating School Quality

Less than 10 miles from Poplar Grove, Annesdale is a beautiful, relatively affluent small city (population is about 40,000) that has two charming city centers filled with restaurants and high-end shopping. According to the

U.S. Census, the median home value is lower than Poplar Grove's, yet well above the county and state average. As in Poplar Grove, more than a few waterfront homes are listed at prices nearing $1 million (at the time of our fieldwork). But Annesdale, where 50% of residents are homeowners, also has a substantial population of apartment-dwellers, including low-income renters who occupy a handful of subsidized housing complexes. This is a serious contrast: in Poplar Grove, 90% of residents own the homes they live in, and apartments and hotels are basically nonexistent (trust us, we checked). On paper, these stats check a number of "desirable" boxes favoring Poplar Grove. Still, the difference is nowhere more glaring than in the "desirability" of schools.

Annesdale High School (AHS) is in the same school district as PGHS, but it ranks in the Top 100 for the state compared to PGHS's Top 10 ranking. In fact, AHS is so much further down the rankings that it's hardly used as a comparison for PGHS (Poplar Grovians sometimes referenced rival Binghampton High as a "good" school, but Sarah and Erica were the only ones who compared AHS to PGHS). And yet both PGHS and AHS have similar numbers of full-time educators who meet state certification requirements—an impressive 99% for AHS and 100% for PGHS—and similar class sizes—both below the state average. But PGHS does have a higher percentage of teachers with more than three years of experience (about 90%, compared to 70% at AHS) and a lower counselor-to-student ratio (about 225 students per counselor, compared to 300 per counselor at AHS, with the recommended ratio being 250:1). At a school level, PGHS shows some small advantages in terms of what the school can offer students, but none that really helps explain the differences in academic rankings and subsequent reputational differences observed during our time in Poplar Grove.

It's always difficult to compare academic excellence between schools. While the inputs to education—like class size, teacher qualifications, and so on—all matter, academic excellence in the United States is highly associated with characteristics of the student bodies and their families—characteristics like socioeconomic status, parental education, and other forms of privilege. In other words, in the United States, the experiences and resources kids bring with them *to* school are extraordinarily determinative to which youth are able to take advantage of opportunities to learn *in* school.[9] In effect, school statistics like rankings, average SAT scores, and graduation rates are heavily confounded with students' demographic characteristics. Simply put, it is much easier for a school to boast exceptional metrics—to be ranked number one—if the majority of its students are privileged. Annesdale, with its lower rank and much lower graduation rate, may look like an objectively "worse" school, but 40% of the students who walk through its doors are economically disadvantaged (according to National Center for Education Statistics data), compared to *less than* 5% of Poplar Grove students. Annesdale starts the rankings race at a disadvantage.

This is why it is helpful to compare student performance in each school's most academically elite classes—the Advanced Placement (AP) classes. Basically, this approach allows us to hold constant the motivation, academic orientation, privilege, and all other unmeasured *stuff* that enable students to get into those top classes, asking only, once a school's kids are in the AP classes, how do they fare? With the caveat that it is possible it's harder to get *into* AP at Annesdale than at Poplar Grove (schools can have different procedures for entry), an overall higher percentage of students at Annesdale High earn college credit for their AP high school courses than do students at Poplar Grove High. Both schools appear highly capable of educating their most talented, motivated, and likely most privileged students. Educational attainment scholars also agree that distinctions between schools, on average, matter less for the kinds of middle- and upper-middle-class youth who generally call Poplar Grove home.[10-14]

So by the numbers, there isn't anything wrong with Annesdale High. Quite the contrary: by many objective standards, it is a good school. Its relative desirability appears, instead, linked to the community and school's demographic diversity—demographic diversity that makes Annesdale High fall in rankings based on all the students attending the school. So much of what schools can do in terms of producing positive academic outcomes for students depends on the resources that kids walk into the school building with. And Poplar Grove High benefits from working with such an economically secure and privileged population.

Of course, how we evaluated school quality is not how lay people evaluate "good" schools. What we have offered our readers is an evaluation grounded in years of experience researching schools and understanding how schools work. What Harrison and his fellow parents in Poplar Grove did—look at average test scores and school rankings, and use that information to do their best to find a school that will support their child's future—is what many concerned parents try to do around the United States. What goes unspoken is that this process often leads children from the higher socioeconomic statuses to attend racially and socioeconomically homogeneous neighborhood schools. Parents who can choose, choose what looks best to them. And because of how parents in places like Poplar Grove tend to choose neighborhoods based on school rankings, and because school rankings are confounded with students' demographic characteristics (particularly markers of privilege), this individual process of selecting a place to call home and a school to send your kids to can compound collectively to reinforce and even drive the creation of homogeneous communities, whether that was the intention or not.

1.4 THE DARK SIDE OF AN IDEAL COMMUNITY

Why does this matter, you may be asking? How does this relate to our focus on understanding why so many youth die so young and by their own hand in Poplar Grove? Well, as we saw earlier, there is some allure to living in Poplar Grove. This allure is tied to the reputation of the community and the reputation of the local public schools, and it is recognized by insiders and outsiders alike. While this reputation is predicated on the impressive stats of the local public schools and housing prices, the school and community "desirability" is also facilitated by those unnamed privileges that many Poplar Grovians hold: they are largely White and in the upper echelons of socioeconomic status.

Here's why this matters. Protecting reputations can become a really high-stakes game. And we found that this game ultimately had unintended consequences for the parents and children living in Poplar Grove. Parents moved to Poplar Grove looking for a great place to raise their children, not a homogeneous, wealthy enclave *or* a pressure cooker that their kids would struggle to survive. And while the parents we spoke with took for granted that a good way to find a good school for their kids was to use available data on school rank and test scores, they did not appear aware that this would almost certainly result in their children living in homogeneous neighborhoods and attending homogeneous schools. Maybe that wouldn't matter—after all, these kids have a lot of advantages—except that there are downsides to living in homogeneous communities, whether that homogeneity is based on race, ethnicity, socioeconomic status, culture, or a mix of factors.

Most notably, research has shown that homogeneity can amplify the power a community has over its denizens, the power to control what they think and do.[14] That power can be used for good—it helps explain why Poplar Grovians can build and sustain such wonderfully supportive ties within the community. It helps explain why it is so easy to gather a group of moms for morning walks, and why we feel so welcomed by the community when we return. But homogeneity can also create pressures. Some of those pressures may be prosocial and beneficial to most, if not all, members—pressure to be a good neighbor, pressure to show up for a visiting sociologist's latest talk. But others can be unintentionally harmful—at least to some members. Homogeneity and a desire to protect reputations—especially a reputation as illustrious as Poplar Grove's—usually come with pressures to live up to community expectations. This can mean that the slightest differences or deviances from the community's expectations can become painful.

Homogeneity in a community can also distort the everyday choices parents make while raising their children—like expectations for children's grades or ideas about pathways to prosperity in young adulthood. What is actually a choice can become a taken-for-granted social fact that steers community members toward protecting the community's reputation for excellence rather than the particular needs of their child. And all without the parent or child necessarily noticing.

We will spend the rest of the book unpacking these consequences of life in this beautiful, idyllic, homogenous community. Because we did find that the very forces that made Poplar Grove such a warm and caring community could also render it an exhausting place to live. But before we move onto that, let's discuss the final element of connectedness in Poplar Grove and how those connections work to maintain Poplar Grove's impressive reputation.

1.5 THE GOSSIP MILL

Anyone who has lived in a small, tightly knit community can probably anticipate one of the main ways that reputations are guarded in communities like Poplar Grove. Many Poplar Grovians referred to the community as being home to a very well-developed and active "grapevine." Shara, a young adult we met, shared, "[Poplar Grove's] a huge gossip town. Everyone knows your business." While gossip is easy to judge as tacky or distasteful from a distance, let's be honest: We all do it at one point or another. It's just a fact of community life, found everywhere from extended families, academic departments, high schools, and communities like Poplar Grove. In many ways, gossip is essential, representing perhaps the oldest form of informal social control—or the pressure to control people's behaviors so that they fit within expectations.[15,16] Gossip helps keep people in line. People gossip to remind others of their place—sharing their assessments of others' actions and subtly, or not-so-subtly, reinforcing the community's preferred social norms. Even the threat of gossip is functional.[17] Under just the threat of gossip, group members will self-regulate their own behaviors, lest they become the topic of gossip themselves, reaping embarrassment, shame, or ostracism. In other words, gossip is central to protecting individual and collective reputations.

In Poplar Grove, where achievement and affluence blend together to form powerful expectations, gossip is truly stressful. "We have lived here, in this house, for 20 years, 22 years, and we don't have a lot of friends," Diane, a mother, told us. "This woman right next door . . . There used to be a time when I used to go on walks with her, when my daughter was a baby and she had a baby. And you know what? All she was doing was gossiping! It was just gossip talk, I barely say hi to her anymore; [she's] just a big mouth who thrives on that kind of stuff, you know? And there is a lot of that here."

To be sure, a lot of Poplar Grove's gossip is benignly judgmental, the status-seeking normal to affluent communities: people might comment on what someone wore to the grocery store. However, a lot of the gossip was centered on accomplishments—specifically, children's accomplishments. And this is where things could get a bit dicey for kids. Victoria, mother to self-described "ideal Poplar Grove teen" Shannon, labeled Poplar Grove a "share-and-tell-and-showoff" type of town. Indeed, parents and youth reported hearing gossip about kids' GPAs, college admissions, and athletic achievements in the stands at sporting events and at social events like cocktail parties. Parents anxious about children being admitted to the "right" colleges, earning scholarships and accolades, become more anxious with every conversation, said Adalyn, a parent: if "you just stand around [at parties] and listen to conversations, you can hear stuff like" parents bragging about setting up video cameras to "record their child's on-field performance" for college admissions. Everyone here seems to know they are being watched and evaluated, their lives exposed and dissected by their fellow residents.

It's already an off-putting thing to realize a community weaponizes information and invades privacy for the sake of status-seeking and to ensure expectations are both widespread and obeyed. But in the context of Poplar Grove's recurring suicide losses of youth, the grapevine could be even darker.

Echoing Diane's decision to opt-out of the rumor mill, Victoria said, "I had this one girlfriend where I basically had to shut her down, 'cause

I'm not good at sharing other people's information." She emphasized, "If it's not my information to share it, I'm not gonna do it, and I wish people would respect that in *all areas*." It turned out her aversion was closely linked to the town's youth mental health crisis.

Victoria is close to the family of one of the more well-known youth who died by suicide, Quinn. She tried hard to protect her friends, Quinn's parents, from the gossipy details flying around town. To her, it felt like the grapevine wasn't acting "out of sympathy," but because it gave its participants a form of power. Indeed, detailed knowledge about suicides spreads incredibly fast in Poplar Grove. The day after Michelle died by suicide, Diane, the mother we met above, was driving her nephew to an early flight when she got a 5 a.m. phone call from a friend of Michelle's mom. "This is *not a friend*," Diane clarified, but the woman wanted to share the news: "I have some bad news: Michelle hung herself." Cryptically, the caller warned Diane to "watch out for your daughter," a confusing comment that left Diane yelling into the phone, "What do you mean?! What does that mean?!!" Having implied that perhaps Diane's daughter had a pact with Michelle, the caller added nothing and was off, presumably to make more calls, leaving Diane in terrible distress. Similarly, Quinn's mom Cora remembered an instance when she was chatting with a woman who worked at the gym in the community center: "I can't remember how it came up, but I was talking—'cause she's had a few suicides in her family— and, so we were just kinda talking about it and I guess I said something about how Quinn died, and the lady's like, 'Oh, that's not what I heard, I thought she slit her wrists.'"

The detail of the gossip was often shocking, though it blended truth and hearsay. We heard conflicting stories from interviewees, for instance, about PGHS graduate Brian's death by suicide, with some saying the young man suffered from mental illness and others, including his parent, citing Brian's struggles with meeting expectations. More often, and more unsettlingly, though, the gossip was intimate and extraordinarily accurate. A good example came from a parent named Margaret. She told us she did not know Emmett—who died by suicide—or his family well, but "heard through the grapevine [that Emmett] . . . was in and out of a mental institution a couple of times, is what I understand." She continued, sharing that she heard Emmett

> had counseling, he had threatened many times . . . The last fight [he had with his parents] was, "You're getting really bad again, I think it's time for you to go back to the hospital," and that's when he hung himself. That's the rumor I heard. It's qualified, but it's still a rumor.

Shockingly, we corroborated many of these details in our own conversations with people who were close to Emmett. The teen had been in and out of the hospital; he'd had counseling; and he had experienced suicidal ideation prior to ending his life. That Margaret, a person with no close ties to Emmett or his family, knew all of these private, painful details of Emmett's story is illustrative of a pattern in Poplar Grove. The reality is that these stories are floating around in elaborate detail for community members to casually pick up and dissect.

Ultimately, tight-knit communities offer support and security often lacking in larger, more impersonal urban spaces, and yet these same tight-knit communities also facilitate the gossip that makes it easier to know the private details of other people's lives and monitor other people's behavior. There was a constant threat that people's privacy would be violated. People in Poplar Grove want to "have a picture-perfect family," in the words of a young adult named Hillary, and gossip offered anecdotal warnings of what happens when families or kids stray from expectations. This creates pressure to conform. Within Poplar Grove's overlapping social relationships, status-norms of affluence, and homogeneity, everyone can easily identify (and identify with) everyone else. All of this raises the stakes for not fitting in.

1.6 CONCLUSION

Poplar Grove was not what we expected to find when we arrived in the community, knowing only its location and that it was home to an enduring

youth suicide problem. Poplar Grovians were quick to tell us—and then
to show us—how much they helped each other out, how they took care to
support each other and each other's children. Almost everyone we spoke
with reported what a wonderful place this was to raise a family and to
grow up in. The intense community orientation was, we found, in many
ways quite deliberate. It was supported by community organizations and
neighborhoods that included beautiful shared public spaces—parks,
pools, beaches—that made gathering and socializing with neighbors easy.
Poplar Grovians can just walk out their backyards into shared spaces filled
with kids and parents ready to play or chat. This powerful sense of community draws young adults back to raise their own children in the illustrious schools and along the soothing banks of the community's rivers.
Between the ethos of social support, the tight-knit safety net, and the enduring intergenerational web of social relationships, Poplar Grove *is* an
inviting place.

So why, then, is Poplar Grove also the site of a smoldering adolescent
suicide problem that has snatched away a disproportionate number of
those kids over more than two decades? We began to find the answer in
Poplar Grove's reputation as the most elite community in the local area.
People were drawn to Poplar Grove not only for its wonderful sense of
community; they were drawn there for the top-ranked schools and the
"desirable" neighborhoods. Kids saw it as almost a given that to live in
Poplar Grove, you have to be affluent. And the affluence in Poplar Grove
served to further demarcate it from surrounding communities. Many
want to be a part of Poplar Grove, but not everyone can afford the price of
admission. This was also evident in the tangible material goods—the cars
in parking lots, the clothes people wore—in Poplar Grove. While we did
not find any of the people we met in Poplar Grove "snooty," kids understood the external perception of their town to be the "rich," moneyed area.
And while we doubt Poplar Grovians would argue that makes them better
than other people (in fact, they'd likely emphatically counter that statement), living in an intensely sought after, desirable community has certain consequences. It puts pressure on people to maintain Poplar Grove's
reputation. It puts pressure on people to conform to social expectations

not just to be caring, good neighbors, but also to fit into certain expectations for what it means to be a Poplar Grovian. This pressure is further amplified by just how homogeneous the community is—in terms of race and ethnicity, along with socioeconomic status—particularly since Poplar Grove is surrounded almost on all sides by more diverse communities. We know from existing scientific research that being surrounded by people who are "like us" can amplify identification with our group of similar others and intensify distinctions between in-groups and out-groups. And everyone wants to be "in" in Poplar Grove, and the boundaries for falling out are proximate.

Not surprising to anyone who has ever lived in a small community, we found these boundaries—between in and out—to be reinforced in everyday interactions, namely through gossip. People talked, and private, personal information was shared. This meant that everyone in Poplar Grove lived under the threat of losing their privacy. Fitting in mattered, and if you didn't, your neighbors were sure to find out.

In short, this beautiful, connected community rich in social support had some challenges built into the very same tightly woven fabric of community life. In the next chapters, we'll explore how this social fabric contributed to Poplar Grove's suicide problem. It is exactly that connectedness, so often seen as a positive social good, that can at times be toxic and problematic to children and families' well-being.

REFERENCES

1. Lynd RS, Lynd HM. *Middletown: A Study in Contemporary American Culture.* New York: Harcourt, Brace, and Co.; 1929.
2. Wuthnow R. *The Left Behind: Decline and Rage in Rural American.* Princeton, NJ: Princeton University Press; 2018.
3. Collins R. *Interaction Ritual Chains.* Princeton, NJ: Princeton University Press; 2004.
4. Lareau A. *Unequal Childhoods: Class, Race, and Family Life.* Berkeley: University of California Press; 2003.
5. Hechter M. *Principles of Group Solidarity.* Berkeley: University of California Press; 1987.
6. Strauss AL. *Mirrors and Masks.* Glencoe, IL: The Free Press; 1959.

7. Adelman R. The Role of Race, Class, and Residential Preferences in the Neighborhood Racial Composition of Middle-Class Blacks and Whites. *Social Science Quarterly*. 2005;86(1):209–228.

8. Owens A. Racial Residential Segregation of School-Age Children and Adults: The Role of Schooling as a Segregating Force. *RSF: The Russell Sage Foundation Journal of the Social Sciences*. 2017;3(2):63–80.

9. Calarco JM. *Negotiating Opportunities: How the Middle Class Secures Advantages in School*. Oxford, UK: Oxford University Press; 2018.

10 Blau PM, Duncan OD. The Process of Stratification. In: *The American Occupational Structure*. New York: Free Press; 1967:163–206.

11. Lauen DL, Gaddis SM. Exposure to Classroom Poverty and Test Score Achievement: Contextual Effects or Selection? *American Journal of Sociology*. 2013;118(4):98.

12. Levy BL, Owens A, Sampson RJ. The Varying Effects of Neighborhood Disadvantage on College Graduation: Moderating and Mediating Mechanisms. *Sociology of Education*. 2019;92(3):269–292.

13. Haller AO, Portes A. Status attainment processes. *Sociology of Education*. 1973:51–91.

14. Coleman JS. Social Capital in the Creation of Human Capital. *American Journal of Sociology*. 1988;94(Supplement):S9–S120.

15. Goffman E. *The Presentation of Self in Everyday Life*. New York: Anchor Books; 1959.

16. Shibutani T. Reference Groups and Social Control. In: Rose AM, ed. *Human Behavior and Social Processes*. Boston: Houghton Mifflin Company; 1962:128–147.

17. Bell MM. *Childerley: Nature and Morality in a Country Village*. Chicago: University of Chicago; 1995.

2

GREAT EXPECTATIONS

We first met Carrie in the chaotic food court of a shopping mall in Frederick, about an hour's drive from Poplar Grove. It felt like an odd choice for an interview about suicidal despair and loss, until Carrie explained, with a laugh, that she figured there was nowhere more anonymous than a crowd of total strangers. We conceded the point: anonymity was in short supply in her hometown, where everyone knew and kept tabs on everyone else.

Like other interviewees, Carrie underscored how exhausting life could feel in the fishbowl environment of Poplar Grove. "When I lived there, I didn't necessarily feel comfortable just going to the store looking like crap. 'What if I run into somebody?' Not that I overly care about my looks or what people think of me, but it just sort of—that's just how it was. You just always just had it in the back of your mind, 'Who am I going to run into? What are they going to think of me?'" Though she had the money to do it and plenty of encouragement from her parents, Carrie decided *not* to call Poplar Grove home in young adulthood. She wanted to put down roots somewhere new, somewhere she could blend in, where there wasn't all the constant pressure and competition she felt growing up.

"We all really wanted to be successful," Carrie remembered of her Poplar Grove High School (PGHS) peers. She said the adolescents internalized all the pressures that permeated the town and spoke of the constant sense of falling behind in the quest to keep up with (let's be real, to out-do) the Joneses. "I wanted to do good in school and I wanted to do great in lacrosse. I wanted to be [Student Government] president . . . I just constantly pushed myself." In fact, she'd achieved all her high school goals. She *was* student government president and lacrosse team captain, and she *was* great at school. She also ended up in the hospital. What her doctors later identified as depression escalated into a suicidal crisis, but Carrie did not reach out to any of the loving and supportive people in her social networks. Feeling utterly isolated, this high school superstar attempted to die by suicide.

Though Carrie's story is deeply personal, it is also enormously instructive because, in Poplar Grove and so many other small towns, the personal tends to reflect the collective experience. As we seek answers and solutions to the enduring youth suicide problem in community-minded Poplar Grove, we must ask what it means to be a kid in this town. What is it like to be raised in a paradoxical town known as much for its shared values, privilege, and close-knit, multigenerational community as for its concentrated tragedy? Looking at the social forces that pattern a Poplar Grove childhood and how they are experienced by kids themselves, we believe, is another key piece of the puzzle. It draws us closer to understanding our core question—why do so many youth in this wonderful community end their lives in suicide?

2.1 A CULTURE OF EXCELLENCE

As we noted in Chapter 1, Poplar Grove's reputation was deeply tied to the local public schools. Known statewide for their purportedly singular academic excellence, it is not surprising that maintaining the excellence of the schools was a core community value. Still, the clarity and consistency with which Poplar Grovians could name their shared values was sometimes uncanny. "We" was a constant refrain. "When we think of Poplar Grove," Elizabeth, a mother of a teen, shared, "We think of achievement, we speak of scholastic achievement, and we speak of sports achievement." Douglas, a school-based mental health worker, concurred:

The expectation and the performance of students at Poplar Grove High School and the whole cluster [of schools] that [feed] into Poplar Grove [High] has been one of athletic excellence, academic excellence: "*We are Poplar Grove, and we are going to achieve!*"

Like Carrie, *all* the youth and young adults that we spoke with in Poplar Grove possessed a clear understanding of these high expectations. Teenager Hadley said, "Like, we are *known* for having the high-level high schools. We're *known* for having some of the hardest curriculum and some of the best turned-out students." Madison and Lily, Hadley's contemporaries, laughed in a focus group over what they called their school's "tagline": "A Tradition of Excellence." In a mocking imitation—perhaps of a teacher, parent, or imagined observer—Madison called out, "Oh, Poplar Grove! *A Tradition of Excellence!* 'Oh, you got a B minus?! What's wrong with you?! Where's your tradition of excellence? I only want to see A pluses!'"

As noted earlier, these were not solely external expectations imposed on youth by adults. Academic and athletic excellence had come to be deeply held internal values among adolescents. As Samantha, a PGHS graduate, explained, the social currency of cool was measured by racking up perfect grades, passing Advanced Placement (AP) exams, amassing trophies and athletic championships. Lily told us it stared earlier: "Going to Poplar Grove Middle School, I feel like a lot of people were pressured to get Honor Roll and Principal's Honor Roll, and a C was bad." With a slightly uncomfortable laugh, she referred to the "academic mentality" and competition she perceived in early adolescence: "GPAs have been, like, a really standard thing people use to compete with each other, and *Standard* versus *Honors* and *Honors* versus *AP* [courses] and everything."

We noted how often youth spoke of these academic hierarchies, attaching pride or shame to taking—or not taking—standard, AP, and honors classes. Molly, a young adult, recalled that "if you, like, didn't take the AP option—and I took an honors option, I felt, like, stupid for being in an honors level instead of in the AP classes." Her contemporary Gwen revealed how she had hidden from her peers a string of Cs in math that caused her to shift out of an AP class: "I didn't tell anybody that I was taking standard [math] because I was terrified that people were going to think, like, so much less of me." In fact, it was clear Gwen had thought less of herself on this measure: "Because, like, when people think—well, until I got into a standard class *I* thought it was going to be, like, burnout kids or kids who just don't give two craps about their education." A third former PGHS classmate, Ander, confirmed the prevailing sentiment: "If you're in your junior or senior year and you haven't been taking APs, *why not? What are you doing?*" Though these young adults were a few years past their high school days, they spoke with awe about their class valedictorian, who they remembered as having taken 19 AP classes.

Keeping secrets about perceived failures was also a theme in these interviews. Even getting a B—which your authors would like to point out (perhaps in their own defense) is an absolutely solid, respectable grade—carried shame. "Like, I had four Bs on my report card, and I was *mortified*," cringed teenaged Natalie. "And I did not want to tell my friends about my grades, because *everyone* is a straight-A student." In their tiny, tight-knit community, though, these were daily topics of conversation. Current and former students revealed the hallway chats and whispers in which kids gossiped about their peers' academics. Natalie had plenty of experiences with kids "who will be really open about [saying] 'oh my gosh, you're so stupid if you aren't like, in Honors Algebra 2 as a freshman.'" Samantha, too, shook her head over similar exchanges at school:

> "Oh, it's classroom registration time, how many APs are you taking next semester? Oh, it's sports transition time, what team are you joining next semester? Oh your team went to the championships, did you place first? What position did you play?" . . . [T]hose are all very normal conversations.

Of course, the grades and AP classes and varsity championships were not the end-goal for Poplar Grove's kids, just steps along the way to the long-term goal of adult success and the replication of their own privileged childhoods for another generation. In that progression, going to college (especially a top-tier one) was a taken-for-granted next step—as recent graduate Vanessa mused in words much like Ander's, "If you're not going to college, what are you doing?"—and kids mainly understood high school as preparation for success at the next level. Elisha, a college freshman, expressed a sort of gratitude that PGHS graduates are "ready for college . . . we're pushed so hard . . . but it, like, definitely prepares us for the college world, too."

Students and adults shared an understanding that college admissions, especially at selective universities, demand well-rounded and highly involved applicants. Not surprisingly, then, we found that being an ideal Poplar Grove student required class-leading academics, extraordinary involvement in extracurriculars, and the "something extra" that admissions teams were seeking. Whether we were interviewing a teen, young adult, parent, mental health worker, or school staffer, these were listed almost verbatim anytime we asked about life in the Poplar Grove community. For Vanessa, living up to the PGHS standard meant "you had to be good at your academics, and you had to be good at some kind of sport, and you had to be good at some kind of arts . . . theater or, like, drawing and painting, or music or something."

What added intensity to this whole college business was that, ideally, kids' high achievement would result in admissions to top colleges that included athletic or academic merit scholarships. As outsiders, the consistency with which parents mentioned the desire for their children to receive a college scholarship was fascinating. In a relatively wealthy enclave, where kids rarely wanted for anything, scholarships were widely emphasized. And while college has grown enormously expensive—making scholarships necessary for more middle-class kids—it was also apparent that scholarships were a deep source of pride and tangible, external validation for Poplar Grove parents—undeniable evidence that their child really was exceptionally *excellent*. Indeed, in this community where most everyone was successful, Heather, a local mental health worker, described the parents and kids as engaged in a "huge competition," in which "their kid [getting] that scholarship to that great college" was a means of setting their family or their kid apart from the crowd. Being recognized as meritorious in athletics or academics was the external status marker that could be—and was—boasted about on Facebook, in the stands at athletic events, or during the PGHS high school graduation ceremony. "Everyone [is] always like, 'Who's getting recruited where?'," Jack, a young adult from Poplar Grove, noted. Amelia, a teen, concurred: "Parents are always posting on Facebook 'Oh! My kid got into this school with a scholarship!'"

By now, we could see that the relatively short-term goals of high school achievement and going to college were part of a broader project that involved raising children capable of reproducing, if not exceeding, their parents' socioeconomic status and security. The kids, as much as anyone, understood the clear expectations about who they should be and what they should do during high school and into college, and how meeting those expectations moved them toward a vision of ideal adulthood. Harrison, the dad we met in Chapter 1, ticked off the checklist:

> There is a, a narrative in this community that essentially says, um, "Your kids will have multiple AP classes, have a high GPA, excel in a sport, excel in drama, um, get a scholarship to Princeton, marry their college sweetheart, end up having a house on the water, two SUVs and a jet ski, oh, and a beach condo." That's the motif. You know, that's sort of, everything sort of moves in that direction.

Importantly, youth in Poplar Grove could look around and see many examples of this good life. To them, the dream of two houses, prestigious jobs, the whole package, was tangible. If their own family didn't have a vacation home, their friends' families did, and they likely tagged along on weekend getaways, fishing, boating, and goofing around in style on nearby waterfront properties. In many cases, parents had explicitly moved to Poplar Grove so their kids could enjoy the advantages of this very social context. This place exemplifies what sociologists call "tight" culture, or a culture where expectations are clear and narrowly defined, without a lot of variation or flexibility.[1] The ties that generate the strong sense of we-ness, of social support and pride in the place also generate this tight, homogenous local culture in which everyone knows exactly who they are supposed to be, how they are supposed to behave, and what they should be doing.[2]

2.2 THE FEASIBILITY OF EXCELLENCE

Against the pervasive cultural directive to achieve, there is a shared sense in Poplar Grove that all the community's children are academically gifted—after all, their parents almost universally hold high-status occupations—and thus academics should come easily to them. Proud mom Victoria half-joked, "If we put [the average kid from Poplar Grove] in the middle of Indiana, [they'd] probably be a rock star."

And the examples abounded. That there absolutely *were* students who embodied Poplar Grove's great expectations only made this exceptional attainment seem more reasonable and feasible. Carrie, from this chapter's opening, was described by a peer as "one of . . . the popular girls who seemingly had all of her shit together and [was a] beautiful, absolutely stunning girl," and that she had achieved all her goals. Shannon, too, understood the assignment and was happy to report she was doing a great job fulfilling it: "I don't wanna sound cocky, but I tend to be exactly what the Poplar Grove ideal is. . . . Like I said, I'm in [student government], team captain, varsity sport . . . but I still go out every single weekend." Her mother and plenty of other students affirmed: delightfully gregarious with long, straight, blond hair and the good looks girls particularly noted were crucial to meeting community ideals, and Shannon got straight-As, captained one of the most prestigious PGHS teams, participated in student government and academic extracurriculars, and in her "spare" time, volunteered with her church group. She'd already been recruited to play her favorite sport at an elite, Division I college. *And* she was popular.

Shannon's comment about going out every single weekend is also relevant. In one more twist to the local cultural expectations, youth were expected to make their achievements "look easy," to succeed *effortlessly*. In a youth focus group, when Beth characterized the "ideal person," adding "if it's, like, hard for you, you don't want to admit it," she was met with a chorus of agreement. The other youth in the focus group nodded along as she elaborated, "Because you look at other people, and you're like, 'Oh, they're doing all this stuff, it must be easier for them,' and then you're like, 'Why isn't it easy for me?'"

In Poplar Grove, success takes hard work. If you can't hack it, it's your own fault. The shared understanding is that the best are the best because they don't struggle to get the top grade, to take the top classes, to be the top athlete. At the same time, perhaps paradoxically, failure to make the grade or to take the hard classes is interpreted not as a lack of talent, but as laziness or the unwillingness to do what it takes. Again, we return to the words Ander and Vanessa, and so many others, used as they recalled the judgments leveled at peers who didn't take AP classes or go to college: *"What are you doing?"* The contradictory messages and obvious binds felt irreconcilable to us as outsiders, and they seemed to have been painful for many young people. Youth were supposed to perform both hard work and ease, to be naturally, effortlessly talented as well as driven to do whatever it took. Performing only one was insufficient if you wanted to fully live up to Poplar Grove's ideals.

2.3 TEENAGE NIGHTMARE

It is not difficult to anticipate some of the downside of the tight and broadly shared culture of excellence that permeates Poplar Grove. Carrie's was just one of many stories in which external pressures became harmful internal pressures. "We're pushed so hard," said Elisha, a recent PGHS graduate, "I guess it's, like, so helpful, but it makes high school very stressful." Though no one was physically twisting their arms or threatening them, many of these young people described their dread, anxiety, and fear regarding the consequences of failing to exceed expectations. Lily, the teenaged focus group participant, explained,: "From the beginning of middle school, we start thinking about a career path." She continued:

> I think that's really hard . . . especially for me, personally. I have no idea what I want to do when I grow up, and from that time, most of your classes and teachers are thinking, "Oh, what are you going to be? What are you going to do? How are you going to make any money? How are you going to support your family? You *are* going

to have a family, right? Blah, blah, blah, blah, blah." I feel like a lot of kids feel like they don't know where they're going, so they're not going anywhere. And then, they realize that there is so much pressure around them that maybe they'll never get out of the pressure, or the *town*, and they'll never get a real job, or a real life outside of their teenage nightmare.

For Lily, the clear picture of what her future *should* look like only highlighted what she didn't know and what she felt she wasn't doing. These fairly normal aspects of adolescent development felt, in her experience, like aberrations and failures. Madison, Lily's contemporary, felt similarly. "I know that a lot of kids feel really stressed," Madison shared, "because even if it's not their parents telling them to do good, it's their teachers and the school and just the environment that they live in, and because it's Poplar Grove! They have to do good, and if they don't do good, they're basically a failure in the eyes of a lot of people."

Madison, like many youth, fluidly flipped between talking about others' experiences and owning those emotional experiences herself. In particular, Madison felt a lot of pressure to fit in and make sure she wasn't "the bottom of the food chain." When she imagined all her peers who were doing better than her, who had more, she'd think, "Like, why aren't I there? Like, what can I do to get there? Why don't I have a job? Why aren't I dating someone? Why didn't I make sports team? I need to try harder."

At the end of every interview in Poplar Grove, we asked whether our respondents wanted us to know anything else, anything we hadn't talked about but was important for us to understand. The pressure was so salient for the younger portion of our interview pool that most said the most important thing we needed to know about growing up in Poplar Grove was the intense pressure to fit into the narrow box of Poplar Grove's great expectations. As we heard in one focus group:

LEAH: Honestly, I just say the most emphasis should be put on the pressure that people feel around here. And even when I try to explain it to my parents, it's hard for them to understand, and it's really hard to explain.

KAITLYN: 'Cause they want what all Poplar Grove parents want.

LEAH: Yeah.

KAITLYN: Their kids' happiness and health and safety.

LEAH: Yeah, but I mean, just the upper-middle class, White people in them, they just don't really realize that it kind of gets old, and it's a lot of pressure. They don't realize how much pressure we put on ourselves as young adults. Some people don't pressure themselves but when kids do, they can be really hard on themselves, especially when they've been kind of raised thinking that they're not good enough.

KAITLYN: Yeah.

LEAH: Not on purpose but that's just kind of how it ends up a lot of the time.

KAITLYN: Yeah, like for example, I spent my summer at the Intelligent Test Prep over there to bump my ACT score up two points with a ridiculous amount of money, so—

LEAH: A *ridiculous* amount of money.

KAITLYN: Like, it's kind of absurd but my parents were gonna make me do it either way, so I was like, "All right, I might as well take the opportunity because I have it." But yeah, it's just kind of crazy because I actually spent five hours a day, three times a week, and it was just—my score went up two points. And then my mom—I got home, and they were like, "Oh, we got your scores back." And then I was like, "Oh my God, oh my God," and then—'cause I just took it, and this happened like three days ago. And then they were like, "Oh, we're really proud of you." And then my—

LEAH: Her dad was like, "There, there." [mimes patting Kaitlyn's head].

KAITLYN: No, my dad was like, "I'm really proud of you, sweetie. You showed a lot of work." And my mom was like, "Yeah, it'd be nice if you got a 30."[i]

LEAH: Which is four points higher than the score that she got! She'd be like, "Yeah, a 30 would be nice."

KAITLYN: Yeah, and I was like, "Don't you think I know that? I was there every day."

LEAH: Yeah, they don't realize that her brain was crying when they said that.

KAITLYN: [Laughs] Yeah, but that's just an example.

ANNA: Yeah.

KAITLYN: And I'm taking it again so—

LEAH: They do it out of love but it's just because, I guess, of the community and the way that parents are, and the expectations and the judgmental adults that do live here. It's just a lot, 'cause even when you're not worrying about your own parents, even when you know your parents will encourage you no matter what you do in life, when you go walking down the street or you go eat dinner at your friend's house, you're worrying about their parents and what they think of you. It's just kind of always there . . . like a subliminal thing.

Certainly, we met many mental health workers, school personnel, medical doctors, and parents who shared teens' perception that the local culture made for a stressful adolescent experience. As Tina, a Poplar Grove mother, shared, "I think it's a wonderful community to raise a family in, and it's . . . great people, but it is very driven. It's exhausting. It's challenging. . . . So, it's kind of a blessing and a curse all at the same time." As early as elementary grades, one school staff member said, the public school system was a "hub of high pressure, high stakes, [and] a very stressful place to be." Another described academic rigor as "crazy."

Despite the value placed on "ease" as youth strive to embody excellence, more than a few respondents spoke about how meeting the expectations for excellence was anything but easy. Georgia, a mother in the community, described PGHS as "very academic" and its staff as pressuring the kids: "They push them, push them, push them to take AP classes . . . It's a lot of pressure . . . If your kid can't figure out [the AP material], like, we've encouraged our kids to do study groups with other kids in the classes. We've had to get outside tutoring. We've used learning centers. . . . It's hard."

Parents often had to activate outside resources, like the learning centers or tutors that Georgia mentions, or expensive athletic club teams that practice in the off-season, often spending significant money in the process. Interestingly, this translates into pressure on parents, too. Their spare time is eaten up by their children's complex schedules and meeting the demands of coaches, principals, and teachers. Tina shared, "You kind of feel like a handler sometimes." She continued:

> You're trying to negotiate between the coach and the teacher . . . we're all on our calendars trying to schedule things, and find some down time, and fun time, and dinners together, but . . . [and as] much as you may not like the system, it is what it is, and you have to kind of operate and play within what you've been dealt. I think that's the frustrating part. I don't think anyone likes it, but what do you do about it?

Tina recounted that one particularly frustrating day her daughter had screamed, "I JUST WANT TO RIDE MY BIKE AROUND THE BLOCK!!!"

"It's sad," Tina concluded, as her fellow parents nodded in recognition. They understood her daughter's frustrated request as emblematic of something larger. The scarcity of leisure afforded these driven kids had become a defining aspect of childhood in the Grove. Louise, a community mother, complained, "We aren't giving our kids permission to be kids." She continued:

> [They're] little shrunken adults. They need to be in all AP classes and you better be doing sports, you better do this, and you need to have it all figured out so that you can get into the right college and you better get into the right college so that you'll get the right job, and I often hear friends say, "Oh, my kids are in this sport, we're scheduled to the hills, we don't have dinner until nine or ten, and we're always eating out." Or, "My kids are up until 1 or 2 o'clock doing homework."

Louise tried to set boundaries:

> I have decided as a parent that that is unrealistic, and we don't do that
> in my house. We're kind of a weird family, and I try not to buy into
> that—I've intentionally not allowed my kids to be in those sports and
> be overscheduled.

Her approach was informed by personal experience:

> I don't like being overscheduled, I hate it when I have something to
> do every single minute of every single day. That squelches my cre-
> ativity; I don't want my children to be that way. I want them to be
> bored, I want them to sit around and not have things to do every
> single minute. And to choose one thing and do it well—you don't
> have to be in five or six activities.

Louise, with her desire for her children to experience boredom, was indeed "weird" in this context. Few parents said they were able to firmly
countermand the local cultural directives, and even fewer kids reported
feeling able to laze about free from the pressure, no matter how carefully
parents tried to help them navigate the intense climate.

At the end of the day, this was quite painful for youth. "It's stressful
being a teenager anyway," Edwin, a clinician with a practice near Poplar
Grove, explained. Edwin thought that the local culture was "[taking away]
some of the fun from growing up" for kids. He and other mental health
workers we spoke with were familiar with the ways this climate created
psychological distress for his clients and their families:

> The message I got over the years [on what makes adolescent life so
> difficult in Poplar Grove] was that it's just this kind of fear of not
> measuring up. . . . They have to do well academically, they have to do
> well athletically, you have to do well socially. I don't know, I mean I'm
> sure you get a lot of that everywhere, but I mean it seems like . . . that's

one of the things kids, adolescents would kind of complain about. You know? They just felt they couldn't quite match their own goals.

Across our conversations with youth, it seemed like Edwin was on to something. Whether the goals are internalized and perceived as being "their own goals" or externalized and perceived as being inflicted on them by the environment, their parents, or their school, nearly every youth or young adult we spoke with felt that the local pressure and cultural expectations caused challenges for their well-being and mental health. The judgment, teen Natalie said, was "kind of hard to escape." She continued:

> There's a lot of, like, not like peer pressures to do things you shouldn't, but peer pressure to fit a certain stereotype. And then you also—like the peer stereotype is that you want to be really popular, and funny, and good . . . like the star of the sports team. But then the parents want you to be this brainiac who is going to go to like an Ivy League school, and I think for some kids that's a really hard fit.

Ultimately, as more and more young Poplar Grovians catalogued a litany of tragic personal consequences, we understood why Lily used the words "teenage nightmare" to describe living under Poplar Grove's overlapping pressures. We heard about hair falling out from stress, "midnight tears" over homework, anxiety, constant worry, insomnia, exhaustion, self-harm, and depression. There were extreme negative emotional consequences attached to "failing" or perceiving themselves to be failing. Gwen struggled with insomnia and, as you'll recall, spoke of being "terrified" that others would think "so much less" of her because she took a standard rather than an AP or honors class. Molly and Carrie called themselves "stupid" for failing to meet their academic expectations. Natalie was "mortified" over getting Bs, and Elisha reported "terrible anxiety" and that high school was about feeling "bad, kind of forever." Theresa, a young adult, described herself as "never good at handling stress in high school," felt "overwhelmed," weathered "midnight tears," and said despairingly, "You can't escape [reality] forever." Samantha spent years struggling with the sinking fear of failure.

Even Shannon, though she declared the pressures had never had any "negative consequences" for her personally, admitted deep concern over feeling like a failure if her team ended their five-year streak as state champions—and characterized it as "not a normal" problem. Failure, in particular, was where emotions got extremely painful and extremely intense for youth and young adults in Poplar Grove. "There's just this sense of pain that comes along with [failure]," Carrie recounted, "it's very personal. It's a reflection on you as a person, that you were not good enough. It's just so internalized and that makes people not want to talk about it, because it's so damning to the person. It's just so deep."

2.4 THE CULTURAL REBELS

Why didn't youth simply reject the local culture? The short answer is found in the narratives of the seven youth and young adults we came to understand as Poplar Grove's "cultural rebels": Scott, Molly, Denise, Chloe, Kaitlyn, Leah, and Avery. They were not unique because of their resilience, nor were they outcasts unable to live up to Poplar Grove's expectations. Most, in fact, embodied many of the local cultural ideals. Instead, they stood out because they refused a whole-hearted buy-in. They saw something wrong with Poplar Grove's culture, sometimes going so far as to say it was "killing kids." As a result, they all made attempts to go their own way and make up their own minds about what it means to be a "good" kid and to live "the good life." The stories they told revealed for us how difficult it really was to throw off the yoke of being a Poplar Grove kid.

Consider, for instance, Scott. Typical of the small cadre of cultural rebels we met, he had one foot in the culture, but was consciously aware that he wanted to keep one foot out. Scott was more sensitive than many of our respondents, and like several of the rebels, he saw himself as "more creative" than, say, academic or athletic. He understood the assignment, as it were, but refused it as often as he could. "I made a choice to break away from the culture and do something that made me happy," he declared. Within his "achievement conscious" community populated by well-paid professional parents and the kids they invested so much in raising to Poplar Grove ideals, he explained, "You have to play a sport. You have to have at least four or five APs." And, he said, you had to equate "success" with "having money" or getting great grades. Instead:

> I made the choice that I wasn't going to force myself to do too much. I was going to do what I needed to do to be happy. I wasn't going to slack off. I was going to do work, but I wasn't going to work to the point of where I would have lost my childhood because you're only young once. I made that decision.

Scott hadn't lost anyone close to him to suicide, but like all Poplar Grove youth, he was aware that it was a huge problem in their community. To him, the culture was harming kids, including him:

> I think it's not a good culture . . . I'm not saying it's bad to get a good education, but there is a certain point where there's that idea that everything is good in moderation. You need to get an education but you also need to make sure you're living life.

Unsurprisingly, he directly tied the cultural expectations to the suicide epidemic: "We are pressured into this, which only adds more pressure and some people can't handle the pressure, [and] *I get this feeling* that a lot of the suicides are because . . . after three or four years of the pressure, they just couldn't take it." He imagined that, when he grew up, "if I start a family, I won't start it here. I would start it in a 'middle of the [road]' neighborhood where they can be children." With a measure of relief, Scott noted that his own parents encouraged him to accept his limitations and focus on being his best self. This surely amplified his ability to resist the local cultural mandates.

And yet, despite Scott's rich analysis of his community and his decision to forge a different path for himself, he shared this poignant reflection:

Sometimes I feel like a lot of people here are going to wake up one morning, *myself included*, and say, "Did it really matter? Does it really matter that I took six APs?" . . . I think *we're* so pressured to achieve that *we've* forgotten that this is, like, one small segment of our entire lives. Ya know? Not that it isn't important. *I know that high school is important and I do get those feelings, like "Oh if I don't pass this test then I'm going to wind up homeless."* I think I don't like that that's the mindset that I go to. I don't like that I have to go to that mindset. *I wish I could change it. I can't.* [emphasis added]

In his comments, Scott reveals that being a cultural rebel is painful, too. It creates a keenly felt dissonance: against his conscious, explicit commitment to rejecting cultural values he finds repugnant, he feels unable to entirely extricate himself from their sway. Deep down, he feels a nagging understanding that this stuff *is* important. As Scott contemplates the consequences of failing an exam, he isn't joking. Though he may be exaggerating a bit with the idea that he could "wind up homeless," he does see the stakes as monumental. Indeed, throughout the interview, Scott presented in various ways. At times, he was confident in his moral conscience and sense that something was amiss in Poplar Grove, but at other times, he presented more timidly, as a youth uncertain whether his read on the situation was right. *What if? What if the culture in Poplar Grove was not local and limited, but the way the whole world worked?*

Ultimately, this understandable uncertainty undermined Scott's protective rejection of the culture and affirmation of his own self-worth. Despite his active project of rebellion, Scott was still enduring the mismatch of his sense of self and Poplar Grove's cultural expectations. For instance, he characterized himself as being "in the lower middle" of the academic pecking order, and told us:

I feel stigmatized. I feel I'm not at the educational level that I should be with everyone else. I should be up there but I'm just not that academic. . . . I'm okay with it sometimes. Sometimes I feel, like, bad about it, ya know . . . Sometimes I wake up in the morning and wonder why I even try, because I know I'm not academic. We are a very academic town. . . . I feel like I'm mismatched. Fish out of water.

Scott's pattern of insightful cultural analysis, rejection of the local culture of academic and athletic excellence (and pressure), *and* difficulty in protecting his sense of self from the local cultural values was emblematic of all of the cultural rebels that we met.

In our small group of cultural rebels, we found two primary (but overlapping) pathways that facilitated their cultural rebellion. The first was paved by caring adults who helped youth make sense of their place in their local cultural environment. Sometimes parents, sometimes mentors, adult rebels were present for Denise, Scott, Avery, and Chloe (and we were able to interview nearly all of these adults, confirming they supported cultural rebellion).[ii]

Like Scott, Denise recognized the cultural expectations to be "perfect," "to [get] all of the grades [and be] amazing at sports," *but* her "totally laid-back California hippie" parents Adalyn and Liam explicitly discussed the harmful culture with her and her sister, Milana. They told the girls, "Don't get sucked into this bullshit drama . . . this is one moment in your life! . . . this is high school. Who cares?!" As a result, Denise shared that she and Milana "tried the best we could to do whatever was expected of us and all that kind of stuff," while feeling very protected from the "constant pressure." Their mother, Adalyn, told us she felt really strongly about the issue: "We make it tough, in [Poplar Grove], for kids to feel like they're okay with themselves. But isn't that a gift that we should all be giving our children when we raise them? You should feel free to feel okay with yourself as a child growing up, whatever that is, that you feel good about who you are no matter what." She continued:

I mean, in this community, parents are too busy to pay attention to their kids and we know that. The kids are here to just bring fame and glory to the family. "Do something remarkable and make us all proud, that's all we care about." Whether it's getting good grades, or having a talent or singing, or on the sports field, or whatever, "That's your job. Your job is to be exceptional and bring fame and glory to the family so that we can brag about you at the cocktail party." There's a big segment of people here that fall into that category.

In response, Adalyn and Liam had tried to turn their home into a haven for youth. They opened their house up, regularly hosting large dinners for any kid that showed up. The meals "lasted two or three hours each night," Denise recounted. "And our friends would flock to the dinner table . . . we talked about . . . what our friends were going through and the pressures that they kind of felt from their parents, and what we could do as their friends to help, and what my parents could do as adult figures in their lives . . . it was very open." Adalyn and Liam walked the walk. When Denise came out, they supported her every step of the way. When she needed mental health help in college, they helped her, nonjudgmentally, with that, too.

And yet Denise and her sister still grew up in Poplar Grove's pressure cooker. There was no way to entirely avoid taking on the challenge of the town's great expectations. "I think it was like our peer group that did it, kind of inadvertently, to each other," Denise explained. "Either someone got pressured from someone . . . or someone's parents [pressured them], and then . . . It's like, 'Oh, well, we've got to keep up' and 'We've got to do all this.'" Indeed, Denise's sense of pride, even honor, was deeply entwined with trying to do the best she could to keep up. It felt wonderful, she said, when her achievements were recognized in the local Poplar Grove paper's Teen of the Week column—a hint of the social emotions like pride and shame that function as moral signals that we are meeting, or not meeting, the expectations of social groups that matter to us. The positive feelings elicited by Denise's community recognition suggest that negative feelings, triggered when she doesn't meet those expectations, still lurk beneath the surface. Perhaps this is why Denise underscored how healthy it was for her "personal development and growth" to choose to move away from Poplar Grove as soon as she could.

Other cultural rebels managed to redefine their sense of what mattered without parents shepherding their way. It was a slightly more painful pathway to cultural rebellion, shared by Molly, Chloe, Avery, Leah, and (by association) Kaitlyn. The key element to this pathway is that these youth lost someone to suicide; it was that experience that triggered their re-evaluation of their adherence to the community's values.[iii]

Molly, a new college student at the time of our interview, would probably offer a shy grin at being labeled a "rebel." Kind, compassionate, and somewhat quiet and serious, Molly was as well versed in the intricacies of being an "ideal kid" as any Poplar Grove teen. Heck, she embodied many of those ideals. She told us academics were "very important" and that she was determined to work hard and get good grades. She played high school sports (though she wasn't on the coveted lacrosse team) and became close with girls in the popular crowd. After graduation, she headed off to a great university. But along the way, she was disrupted by a terrible loss. One of her closest friends, Michelle, died by suicide when Molly was a sophomore in high school. It absolutely rocked her life, setting off years of grief and a fundamental change in her understanding of Poplar Grove's expectations for young people:

> *I think that [Michelle's death] really made me*—it sounds cheesy—but *realize what's important in life*, which is really just your relationships with other people and love and friendship and all that. Because in high school, I was very determined to get good grades. I did, and I worked hard for that, but that was very, very important to me. It still is important, but . . . [now] if I don't get an A in something, that's okay *because I'm still alive. [Grades are] not as important as being happy and having good friendships and relationships and helping people . . .*
>
> *I definitely think that [losing Michelle] has changed the way that I go about school and grades and that kind of pressure.* Not that I don't work hard, *but I know that that's not everything.* To some people, that is everything. To me, it's not. *Because Michelle had perfect grades, but she wasn't happy for whatever reason, whether I knew it or not.* [emphasis added]

Molly's reframing of hard work from something mandatory to something that's "not everything" in the wake of Michelle's death bought her some freedom from stress—something often hard won for kids in Poplar Grove. But like Denise and Scott, Molly also struggled to fully free herself from using Poplar Grove norms as her reference point as she measured her own self-worth. Remember that Molly, in Section 2.1, admitted to feeling "stupid" and ashamed of her "standard" math class, while in another interview, she declared that it was "natural" to get "stressed out a lot about school." She had so fully internalized Poplar Grove's educational norms that they seemed a part of nature, rather than a malleable aspect of culture. Molly and her peers illustrate that it is difficult, if not impossible, for a developing teenager to fully recognize that something they have been taught is obvious, natural, and right is, in fact, malleable, local, subjective, and rejectable.

Cultural beliefs are only as powerful as they are shared and lacking in alternatives.[1] Unfortunately, in Poplar Grove, the great cultural expectations were widely shared, taken for granted as natural and obvious, and because of youth's limited horizons, seemed particularly universal and inescapable. It was hard work to imagine a different world. The cultural rebels helped us understand that rebellion was *possible* and youth were not merely passive receptacles of the local culture, yet fully rebelling against the shared understanding of what it takes to *be a good kid* and *live a good life* was exceedingly tough. Consequently, rather than adopting entirely different beliefs, our cultural rebels lived with a degree of cognitive dissonance. They felt that some things about Poplar Grove were morally wrong, but they also couldn't quite fully reject the local cultural beliefs about good kids and good lives. As a result, every cultural rebel we met was engaged in an iterative, enduring, but ultimately incomplete project of cultural rejection and reframing, presenting as the cliché: you can take the kid out of Poplar Grove, but you really can't take the Poplar Grove out of the kid.

2.5 WHERE DID THE PRESSURE COME FROM?

Before we end our discussion of the local culture in Poplar Grove, it is worth taking a moment to discuss a topic of great interest to Poplar

Grovians during our time there. Where on earth does this high-pressure culture come from? So many parents that we spoke with said—often with frustration—that they didn't grow up this way. Why was so much expected of their children? Others felt absolutely startled that the choice to call this beautiful community home meant taking on a high-pressure status race with the proverbial Joneses. "It's not typical in the places where I lived before . . . all these heavy expectations of bigger and better and best," sighed Maryann, a mother. This led us to witness many conversations focused on who, exactly, was to blame for this culture of pressure, and for the way its stresses accumulate almost invisibly but insidiously into students' distress and, consequently, adolescent suicide deaths. Does this pressure come from high-strung, status-obsessed parents, as some young Poplar Grovians claimed? Or is it the fault of a school system oriented toward high achievement, standardized testing, annual funding renewals, and keeping their legacy of superstar students? Or maybe the more nebulous "peer pressure" is how kids come to recognize and respond to the great expectations they face.

Of all the people we spoke with, young people were the ones who offered the best, and the most accurate, description of where the culture comes from: in short, everywhere. Students blamed parents, the school system, the community writ large, and even each other. Recall Madison's early comment indicting parents, teachers, the school and *"just the environment"* for generating the inescapable pressure. Separately, Hadley used similar terms, telling us the pressure "on kids [comes] from parents, school, and probably, from their peers also." To teens, it appeared the pressure of excellence (or failure) was inescapable and reinforced by all of the major groups of adults that mattered: their parents, their teachers and coaches, school administrators, and random adults they came into contact with (friends' parents, church adults, etc.). Indeed, kids are describing the local culture as working as culture does in most small societies[2,3]: it is co-produced, co-constituted, and co-enforced. Parents, teachers, and kids—each is key to making Poplar Grove the place it is, with all its norms, expectations, and lately, losses. It is worth unpacking how parents and school staff, as the adults with more power than kids (and potentially less insight into the pain this pressure causes), play their roles. We turn first to the role of parents in the production of the pressure culture.

2.5.1 Parenting and the Production of a High-Pressure Culture

Most of the parents in Poplar Grove are professionals with high-status careers. Their skills and practices as successful lawyers, doctors, and CEOs are easily translatable into aspirational skills by which youth can gain success in school. Hadley made this point to explain the academic pressure, using her friend Olivia's family as an example:

> Both of her parents are engineers . . . And they want her to be them. Like they want her to be really good at math, they want her to be in, like, Calculus B/C even though she's in pre-calculus. And, so I think that's where she gets a lot of stress, and what she has to do when she gets older, even though that's not what she wants. I think parents here are crazy, and they try to live through their kids, and they try to push their ideals on their kids for what they want.

In this group, the parenting styles that contribute to the culture of pressure can feel pretty natural for parents: successful parents try to identify why they got ahead and teach their kids to do the same.

One way that elite parents across the United States work to produce excellence in their children is by engaging in a very child-centered, intensive form of parenting aimed at maintaining the child's competitive edge in society. To give their child every advantage, parents actively structure children's lives (especially outside school) so they are full of enriching activities designed to optimize education, development, and opportunities for future advancement. Parents who engage in this style of parenting are often called "helicopter parents"—or, in Poplar Grove, as one parent joked, "B52 Bomber parents." If you happen to read a fair amount of sociological literature, you may know this style of parenting as "concerted cultivation."[4,5] It is a widespread form of parenting among middle- to upper-class US parents. Earlier, Tina, a Poplar Grove mother, alluded to this style of parenting when she mentioned how stressful and exhausting raising kids in Poplar Grove could be. "I don't know that this is just Poplar Grove, as much as it is . . . the socioeconomic class that we're in," Tina reflected, "but [kids here are] very scheduled. . . . We're just on the go, go, go all the time. . . . We spend a lot of time moving from activity to activity, and even our fun is scheduled, so it's kind of a 'rat race.'"

While it can appear "natural" for parents to want to maximize their children's development and secure their futures, it is not, however, consequence-free. Children raised this way have little free time—just like their parents, who end up frantic and time-pressured getting their kids to all the appointments, lessons, training sessions, camps, and activities. Kids can lose out on learning how to amuse themselves creatively, to try out (and even discard) new activities on a whim, and simply relax and be kids.[5] Indeed, finding time to just be a kid wasn't easy. Recall what Tina shared earlier: her daughter had to result to screaming to just be allowed to ride her bike for a bit.

Mental health workers and educators in Poplar Grove also recognized concerted cultivation as the defining characteristic of the local parenting culture. Connie, a mental health provider, reported, "Parents are passionate about their kids to a fault. In many cases . . . I suppose that . . . the Poplar Grove parents, to a great extent, fit the hovering helicopter parent model that people talk about." She continued:

> We've [in my clinic] been really surprised to see, to hear stories like the father that goes over to his son's school that's about to get a 'B' in an AP class and says, "He needs to drop this because he can't afford to get a 'B' in [an] AP class" because he's going to go wherever he's going to go—Princeton, Yale, Harvard . . . mostly I would say there is this protection that goes on. They don't want the kids to hurt in anyway. They don't want them to be disappointed or deprived, or they just don't want them to feel bad. And so it's all very loving and well-intended. . . . But lots of protection, lots of protection and

making sure that [the children] get involved in as many activities as possible so that the options stay open for their lives.

Perhaps ironically, being protective, caring parents in this way ends up reinforcing the notion that grades are critically important. As is admission at a top, elite university. The only way out of an AP class for some kids in Poplar Grove requires they get further entrenched in the high-pressure culture. Whether parents actively worked to raise the standards of excellence in the community or moved into Poplar Grove's ready-made culture and adopted it (however hesitantly) or simply did what everyone else was doing (so far as they knew or believed) or even tried to rebel, the culture of achievement and pressure enveloped them as surely as it did the kids. No parent wants to put their kid in a compromised situation, nor do they want to see their child not fitting into a cherished community. Most parents were in a sort of trap of their own design: high-achievers themselves who love their kids, are often proud of them, and want the best for the kids they are raising in a relentless culture of excellence.

Importantly, it could be hard for parents to recognize their own role in the production of academic pressure. Helen's dual roles in the community—as a mental health worker and a mother of three—gave her a status that afforded her a unique sensitivity and reflexivity few other respondents could cultivate. Through her job, Helen had to work with parents and children. Helen shared, "I look at some parents [at my practice] and I go, 'Why did you let [your child] take all of these classes?' This isn't who they are. Let's . . . make them successful for *them*." Helen could be quite critical of parents. Her sense was that parents did not erect enough barriers to protect their kids from endless pressure to achieve. In fact, she saw them as complicit in pushing youth. Applying that perspective to her own parenting, she said, meant trying to be a "guide . . . trying to help [her kids] sort out those competing expectations: [those that] are realistic and what expectations aren't realistic." But at the same time, Helen acknowledged that it was sometimes hard for her to resist pressuring her own children. Helen, of course, was a highly successful professional who had the respect of many in the community. "As a parent I have high expectations for myself," she admitted, "and I sometimes have to keep myself in check so that my kids don't see that and internalize an unreal set of expectations." Being an antipressure parent in Poplar Grove required substantial effort and insight, and in our experience, most parents did not go that route. Or if they did go that route, their children (who we often also interviewed) did not feel the benefits. They still felt the pressure, often intensely.

This is, of course, because parents themselves were part of a system larger than themselves. Parents' social worlds revolved around their children, and they were judged publicly for their performance as parents. "Being highly involved with what our kids were doing," Harrison reasoned, "[meant] we tended to have our social life, meaning mine and my spouse's, sort of revolve around what the kids were doing." He continued:

> As a result, we would make connections with other parents on the [sport's] sideline. So, from a parenting point of view . . . we know a lot of people because of their kids. As opposed to just adults functioning as adults on some sort of adult-thing, it's more of, "What happened at last week's soccer game?" And so, this cadre of both kids and parents sort of tracks through the school system. So, you see them in the elementary, you see them over at the middle school, uh, and then they get to the high school, and there gets to be some differentiation there as the kids, um, move into sort of whatever area of interest is . . . We spend a lot of time in the football stands and the basketball bleachers, and, again, it's sitting next to those parents.

Youth success was a linchpin in Poplar Grove's strong collective identity—as the number-one school, as the most desirable community—and this was reinforced for parents through the intense connectedness. The pressure was on parents, too; the threat of gossip that concerned youth also impacted parents. It taught them that a good parent keeps their kids properly enriched. The anticipation of social judgment attenuated how parents handled parenting. No one, it appears, was free to just parent as they wanted to parent—free of the web of social ties that both gave their lives meaning and set firm constraints around expected behaviors. In other words, free of the local culture. These successful adults feared being shamed, feared their children being shamed or losing out in the class competition, and feared their families being judged harshly and socially excluded. All this led to some potentially unhelpful behavior. "I think it is hard for people to admit," Victoria reflected, but "you don't wanna show weakness in front of all these successful things going on in the town. But this kind of thing means that it isn't as great as everybody thinks it is, you know?"

2.5.2 The School's Role in Generating Pressure

Schools' reputations generally hinge on their academic track record, as well as their athletic and extracurricular programs' spirit-building accomplishments. As Shannon's mom, Victoria, noted, standardized testing scores of PGHS students regularly vault them into the 99th percentile. Because this testing determines school rankings (which attract families to school districts and impact property taxes), schools at the top get no chance to rest—they must always keep up standards so they continue to draw students to the school catchment area or risk losing out on ever-scarcer funding. And the community is watching PGHS. Whether the public schools are maintaining their standards was discussed in the local Poplar Grove newspaper, where the principal of PGHS was called upon to defend a tiny slip in rankings that happened shortly after our fieldwork ended. The principal of PGHS countered by presenting stats on student attendance, student plans to attend college, and the percentage of students on the Honor Roll (i.e., the percent of students earning As and Bs). These "paint a truer picture of the high school experience at PGHS," the principal reasoned, a bit defensively.

While we were not able to conduct ethnographic observations at PGHS to see for ourselves the culture of this school, we were able to review school communications posted publicly on their website. During the 2015–2016 school year, for example, the principal's newsletter to parents regularly emphasized academic achievement and the schools' "Standard of Excellence" (just as Madison promised, earlier in this chapter). "We must make sure all of our students are prepared for spring testing," the school administration wrote in one newsletter. "We are very proud of our continued academic success," they shared, after noting the excellent accolades PGHS had received the year prior. In addition to noting the high rank of PGHS, the administration went on to note the percentage of students on the Principal's Honor Roll (all As, 13%) and the Honor Roll (As and Bs, 56%), and named a series of students receiving even more elite academic accolades. It's clear that PGHS, too, understood the assignment. This messaging was absolutely consistent across the months, years, and instances we had to observe PGHS, if from a distance. PGHS actively embraced its reputation of excellence, with pride, and it worked constantly to maintain that status, much like affluent parents engaging in concerted cultivation.

Parents and kids alike were quite emphatic that the school contributed to the emphasis on academics, athletics, and excellence. Helen, the mother and mental health worker from earlier, had strong feelings about the role of PGHS:

> I will give you an example. The [principal] sends out in the first newsletter of the year, "We are expecting all of our students to reach their highest potential, and we will have no blah-blah-blahs average grades, we will all have this." And . . . I said, "Well, this is an inclusion school [meaning kids with learning disabilities or special needs are included in general education classrooms]. How in the world are they going to have 100%?" And he wasn't talking about 100% participation. He was talking about 100%—we're gonna get this [perfect] grade! I said, "That's impossible!" Right off the bat, the parents of the average kids are already [panicked] . . . "What are we gonna do? How are we going to get this? We got to get our kid tutored, we got to do this, we got to do that." Kids don't want to go to tutoring after they've been in school all day long. They want to go outside and play in the front yard! But no, we're not allowed to do that, because . . . they're going to tutoring because their principal says they're going to have 100% on the standardized tests!

While students with learning disabilities or special needs often are provided accommodations to help ensure testing reflects their knowledge,

Helen's interpretation of the principal's message is that it's not enough to just reach your "highest potential," since "no average grades" are allowed. Helen heard a demand for perfection and felt the pressure. Interestingly, she also believes that this message is going to spur parents into action—passing that pressure on to their children, through tutoring and denying access to free time and outdoor play.

Our own read of the principal's newsletter message on testing that matches Helen's time frame is that it did emphasize excellence, maintaining educational rankings, and making sure that "all of our students are prepared" for the battery of tests that are given in the Spring semester (APs, state competency tests, etc.). Though not every quote that Helen mentions appears (admittedly, it's impossible to be sure that we got the exact right newsletter), what is clear across newsletters from this period is that they consistently mention academics, rankings, and the need to maintain excellence. Whether the principal meant to use these facts to communicate a demand for perfection or not, these are the very moments—in communication and interpretation—that the school's role in the production of a high-pressure academic culture can be observed.

Parents and students also reported pressure from the school to take academically challenging classes, and that the school was inflexible and unresponsive to concerned parents. "So, here's what happened," Margaret, a mother we interviewed, shared. "[My daughter] decided eventually that she could move one of these AP classes to her senior year and balance [her junior-year schedule] out a little more effectively," Margaret relayed. "She went to the counselor—who I'm still mad at—went to the counselor and said, 'I want to drop this class.' It was the last day that they could add/drop for the coming year, I guess. . . . And the counselor talked her back into taking the fourth AP, which was a science class. Not necessary for anything, just a little, you know, *bonus*." First, it's important to note that Margaret's daughter, Amelia, tells this story the same way as her mother. "The counselors really push AP classes on you!" Amelia complained. "I had this experience last year when I wanted to drop one of my AP classes, because I was taking four . . . and my workload was just completely overwhelming. It was like a whole big deal, and it took two weeks to get approved . . . I didn't know why I couldn't just say 'I don't want to take four

AP classes.'" Amelia's experience is notable because school counselors play critical roles in mental health safety nets in schools. To the extent that school counselors are used to push academic excellence, they become *sources* of the high-pressure culture rather than trusted adults that kids can turn to when they are suffering at the hands of said culture.

Of course, Margaret's story, as it continues, also reveals how interconnected all of these social actors—the school, parents, peers—are in producing the culture. Margaret continued, explaining what happened when her daughter, Amelia, returned from the school counselor appointment and said that she had signed up for the fourth AP class after all:

> Amelia comes home to me at the end of the day, and I say, "What did you do? We talked about this." She cried, I cried, and she says, "But mom, you don't understand. All my friends—if they can do it, I can do it."

Having internalized the demands of the culture of achievement, courtesy of social comparisons to her peers, Amelia nonetheless spent the summer nervous about the demanding class schedule coming in the fall. Her mother recalled:

> Midway through the summer, [Amelia] turns and says to me, "I can't do it." And so I said, "Okay, I'll get you out of it." So I start calling over to the school in July. I had meetings, I called, I wrote letters back and forth . . . "You missed the date, the county regulations," blah blah blah. Two weeks into school [in the fall], she's still taking the four APs. I'm told "it can't possibly be changed," because she missed the deadline to change it. She missed the deadline because the counselor forced her to miss the deadline, right? "It can't possibly be changed," even though transfer students and everything else have changed their schedules, they can't *possibly* change hers.

When these dogged attempts could not get her daughter's schedule changed, Margaret decided it was time "to play the game." As she told us, "I sent a letter to the principal talking about suicide and depression—it was right on the heels of the last suicide [snaps fingers]—it got changed. That's how you have to play the game here." As her story closed, Margaret returned to the idea of who's to blame for Poplar Grove's pressure problem: "So, it's not me at all times. So, a lot of the times, it's the school."

In a town with a lot of stressed-out kids and a significant, visible youth suicide problem, the school's role in sustaining intense achievement and athletic pressures—and its perceived unwillingness to make changes to mitigate the pressure, distress, and suicide problem—invited intense criticism. Certainly, schools attempting to deflect blame in children's deaths by suicide are often motivated by protecting the institution's reputation and concerns about legal liability.[6] Yet school staff spoke about feeling like they were caught between a rock and a hard place: they'd built the school in the image demanded by parents deeply engaged in concerted cultivation, then were harshly rebuked when the school was implicated as a driver of youth suicide. It is important to note that school staff are often as deeply troubled by student suicides as any other community member, including parents and students. They shoulder the same difficult emotions, including the gnawing fear of suicide clusters. But because school staff felt they were limited in what they could actually do, given competing parental and budgetary demands, they placed the burden of suicide prevention outside their domain.

2.5.3 It's All Intertwined

While we've tried to illustrate the roles that parents and the school play in generating the culture, these forces are deeply intertwined. The battle that could unfold between parents and school staff was one of the saddest—and most frustrating—parts of our fieldwork. Both sides were sometimes intent on blaming the other for their role in the academic pressure and subsequent suicide problem. One evening, after a community event to discuss mental health, Anna observed a standoff between a school staff member and two parents. "You shouldn't count middle school grades towards kids' high school GPAs [even if kids take a high school course in middle school],"[iv] one parent declared emphatically to the school staff member, "it's harming their self-esteem and their GPAs!" The second parent agreed: "It's increasing pressure on middle school students, too. We should put their mental health first!" The staff member, glancing at Anna, and noticeably frustrated, countered, "You all are the parents! Why don't you just teach your kids that GPA isn't everything? They should take the classes that they want and work hard and be satisfied with their grades." The rumble continued for a while, back and forth, with no progress and no empathy or even apparent desire to understand the other person's perspective. Both parties clearly expected Anna to side with them (she didn't weigh in). In truth, the school staff member may not have had the authority to change what grades count for what, since these were classes tied to graduation requirements. That authority likely lies with the district or even the state department of education. But rather than the staff member explaining their rationale, or showing any authentic interest in the parents' concerns, the staff member immediately went to the oldest pattern in the school's play book: it's not our fault; it's parents' fault. Shortly after this exchange, parents staged a pro-mental health protest outside the school. The protest was to counter what they described as the school's apparent lack of concern about student mental health. Bearing signs that said things like "YOU MATTER!" and "YOU ARE LOVED!" parents lined the entrance to the school in an effort, they explained, to try to make sure kids knew that their mental health mattered, that they were more than just the school they went to and their academic accolades.

From our perspective, both sides hold some responsibility. They both play their part in producing the intensely academic culture. And probably neither can change unless they decide to do so together. Rather than focus on who's to blame, on pointing fingers, or on deflecting blame, it would be radically more productive if each could examine themselves, identify the ways in which they place pressure on kids to fit into narrow molds, and then facilitate productive conversations to make change. It can be hard to see our own role. It can be painful, too. But if we listen to Poplar Grove's kids, it's clear that this is what they need the community to do.

2.6 CONCLUSION

The local cultural norms in Poplar Grove are explicit and narrow. All youth are expected to drive toward academic and athletic excellence, matriculate at a first-rate college or university right after high school, and pursue prestigious occupations in young adulthood that will allow them to raise their own children in similar privileged environs—ideally, back in Poplar Grove. What's more, these cultural beliefs were broadly shared. Every single person we spoke with could articulate them, often with a breezy tone that suggested these were the obvious, taken-for-granted social facts of living a good life. Why *wouldn't* you push your children to aim for the stars? Why would you accept anything less than excellence? Of course, this created intense pressure for youth in Poplar Grove, who had to figure out how to meet all of these great expectations while making it look easy. Their classmates did, so why couldn't they?

This pain of social misalignment brought mental health consequences that, on balance, seemed to overwhelm the possible pride of meeting expectations. Yes, the teen years feel dramatic and emotional, but that is partly a function of the ways a teenager's whole life is localized. For these youth, their whole world was concentrated within life in Poplar Grove. These teens grew up being taught that to be from Poplar Grove was an honor and a privilege; they were taught to take pride in their community, an imperative reinforced through the dense networks of social ties and strong sense of community togetherness. Not fitting in was painful. It was hard to not feel the sting of rejection, youth expressed, when they didn't fit the mold. A good number of them engaged in projects of cultural rebellion and took positive steps toward recalibrating their measures of self-worth, yet even the cultural rebels found their self-esteem impacted by the community culture. Particularly when combined with the high degree of social connectedness, this inescapable local culture—which was co-produced by kids with their social comparisons of APs and GPAs, by parents with their concerted cultivation, and by the school with its Standard of Excellence—would have real consequences for families and youth, generating a heightened vulnerability to suicide during mental health crises.

NOTES

i. According to the National Center for Education Statistics, the maximum ACT score the year that Leah took it was 36. Her score of a 26 was well above the state's and the nation's average ACT score for that year and placed her in about the 82nd percentile of ACT scores nationally. According to ACT materials, Kaitlyn's score means she's "ready for college"; however, a score in the 30s may make her substantially more likely to receive financial aid (https://cloud.e.act.org/ebook-a-tool-to-help-plan-your-future).

ii. There were additional parents like Louise, mentioned in the previous section, who reported setting boundaries for their children intended to diminish the pressure, but whose children we did not interview and thus do not know how their parenting impacted their children.

iii. As we said, these pathways are overlapping. Denise also lost a very close friend to suicide, but her pathway to cultural rebellion was fundamentally tied to her parents' support and not the suicide loss (though the suicide loss also made a significant impact on her life).

iv. Quotes in this section are not exact. They are paraphrased from ethnographic field notes.

REFERENCES

1. Martin JL. Power, Authority, and the Constraint of Belief Systems. *American Journal of Sociology*. 2002;107(4):861–904.
2. Fine GA. Group Culture and the Interaction Order: Local Sociology on the Meso-Level. *Annual Review of Sociology*. 2012;38:159–179.
3. Berger P, Luckmann T. *The Social Construction of Reality: A Treatise in the Sociology of Knowledge*. New York: Anchor Books; 1966.
4. Lareau A. *Unequal Childhoods: Class, Race, and Family Life*. Berkeley: University of California Press; 2003.
5. Calarco JM. *Negotiating Opportunities: How the Middle Class Secures Advantages in School*. Oxford, UK: Oxford University Press; 2018.
6. Erbacher TA, Singer JB, Poland S. *Suicide in Schools: A Practitioner's Guide to Multi-Level Prevention, Assessment, Intervention, and Postvention*. New York: Routledge; 2014.

3

WHY YOUTH DIED BY SUICIDE

In my mind, I just can't imagine she's not here.

—Vera

Something about the sheer ferocity of the hug Aria gave her set off Josie's "mom instinct." The family—including Josie's husband Will, brother-in-law Greg, and Josie and Will's other two kids—was already bundled into their SUV for a football game, but there was still plenty of room for Aria. They even had a ticket for her. It wasn't entirely unusual for Aria to opt out like this. Still, Josie couldn't seem to stop texting her middle child after they left for the game. That hug, Josie recalled, felt like, well, like Aria "was never gonna see us again." As Josie said:

> I kept texting her all day like, "Oh what are you doing now?" "Why don't you have your boyfriend over?" Which I never really encourage teenagers to have boyfriends over while no one's home, but I was like [nervous laughter] "Let's get somebody over there!" you know? . . . As soon as she would respond to me, I would send her a different text just to kinda keep her engaged.

Aria, her parents shared, had been a bit "off" recently. Josie and Will had noticed their daughter exhibiting "some of the depression signs," but explained to us—to themselves, maybe—that "it's hard to differentiate it from just being a teenager. You know? You have to get up at 5:30 in the morning; what's wrong with coming home and taking a nap after school?" On balance, the changes they saw in their "upbeat" girl were worrisome without necessarily "rais[ing] red flags." Suicide wasn't on their radar. An idea like that was too terrible, too unimaginable, to really rise up to the level of consciousness. From the car, the football game, all day long, Josie just couldn't stop texting Aria. She needed to.

As it happened, at least two other people were also texting Aria that day. A few doors down, one of her best friends repeatedly reached out: "I'm really worried about you." Her other friend told Aria's mom that her many text messages had gotten no response. Unfortunately, their collective instincts were right; the subtle clues that Aria let slip had been small signals of overwhelming psychological pain. Aria died by suicide that day. The descriptions of the screams that broke out in the neighborhood—when her family came home, when her friends found out—were gut-wrenching. "It's worse than breaking your heart," Aria's uncle Greg said bluntly. "It leaves a hole." Her grandmother Vera described, "It's like there'll always be an empty chair. There's always gonna be a space missing." Losing Aria remains, for all her family and friends left behind, simply devastating.

Though Aria's death came as a shock to much of Poplar Grove, it wasn't a momentary decision. Aria planned her death in advance, documenting her decision in a journal—a handwritten spiral notebook that she titled "The Last 10 Days of My Life." We share pieces of her writing, with her family's permission, so that Aria's perspective and voice may join with the testimonies of her loved ones. And we do so to consider the complexity of each suicide that has brought despair to Poplar Grove.

There was no one "reason" why Aria ended her life. She described herself as "depressed" and "mentally ill," and had told her best friend Katya (but not her parents or, to our knowledge, a clinician) she suspected she had bipolar disorder. Her words ache with a deep sense of worthlessness and how she felt as if "being alive . . . [was] more painful than being dead." Toward the end of the journal, in a letter to her best friend, Aria alluded to the idea that people would be better off without her—a feeling professionals call burdensomeness. As Aria wrote:

No matter how much your smile, laugh, or your goofy personality (my 3 favorite things) could cheer me up instantly, it didn't make me love myself unfortunately. Even when you tried to make me love myself because youre the greatest friend that has ever lived, it didn't make me loathe myself any less . . . I appreciate everything you ever did for me but that only makes me deserve you less. Youre much better off without me, consider yourself set free. Free from my sadness, drama, and problems . . . You're a better person than I ever was and I was only going to bring you down.[i]

Both a sense of worthlessness and a sense of burdensomeness are factors known to be tied to higher risk of suicide.[1] Yet this passage and many others throughout Aria's account also show that Aria loved and felt well loved. She was surrounded by a web of supportive social relationships, and she was fully aware she had them. From a devoted boyfriend to her tight-knit family and adoring friends, Aria had people who were actively trying to make sure she was okay. They took her aside; they asked how she was; they offered help.

In the weeks leading up to her death, parents Josie and Will had spoken to Aria about seeing a therapist. These were not just hollow words—Aria expressed a clear sense that her family or her friends would "save" her, if only she would let them know she needed saving. The journal's entry for Day 6 includes the following:

[My mom is] one of the few that actually knows Im depressed but [she] doesn't know what it feels like first hand. She can detect [my depression] better than anyone too. Im also half honest w/ her because shes my mom and deserves at least some honesty. So I told her how bad Ive felt and she took the time to actually talk to me . . . I felt so loved and she even talked about getting me help. I kinda just brushed it off though. Later that day I had a vision or I guess idea that played in my mind. A vision of how easy it would be to bring this notebook to my mom, tell her Im planning suicide and go straight to a doctor and be saved.

It is also telling that Aria acknowledges, in these pages, that she is important to others and that many people would be hurt by her death. Indeed, it's a major preoccupation of her journal. Her "only doubt," she said of ending her life, "comes from the fact that I how much I would hurt everyone." She is "torn about what to do" because "I [know] how many people I would hurt" by her dying by suicide. These are "people I would never want to hurt in a million years." At another point, we read, "My boyfriend doesn't deserve to be hurt by me like that," and "Same with my mom I dont know if shed ever get over it." One of her final lines in the journal indicates that the purpose of the journal was to convey her feelings—particularly how sorry she was that she had to leave—to the people she was leaving behind:

> Having this notebook was nice so I could write down how I felt my last 10 days but also so whoevers reading knows what I felt. Knows how sorry I am and how much I didn't want to hurt anyone else. This my decision and it's just for the best.

What is so puzzling about a suicide death like Aria's is that while she was, in all likelihood, experiencing significant depression, psychache (or intense psychological pain), and perhaps emergent bipolar disorder (which runs in her family), she was also surrounded by a million and one protective factors. In the end, having caring family and friends with the desire and means to help was not enough to countermand the despair or change Aria's interpretation of how to relieve her pain. Why was a girl who, in her own words "had it fucking made," who understood herself as having her "dream car, 2 awesome parents," who is "thankful for all these things," not able to see her psychological pain and unhappiness as something that could change, that could get better? Why did she interpret her perceived shortcomings as rendering her worthless as a person? *These* are the million-dollar questions, not only when it comes to Aria's death but for the whole community of Poplar Grove. Because this story, of a funny, gregarious, cherished young person, with so much going for them and so many people cheering for them, yet who nonetheless died by suicide, is shockingly common in Poplar Grove.

In this chapter, our goal is to understand why life felt unlivable to a disproportionate number of teens in this community so full of protective factors like having supportive friends and family. How did the mental health safety nets fail so frequently? To develop a social understanding of suicide, we rely on accounts so generously shared both by youth and by the adults in the community struggling to reckon with the so-called suicide epidemic. We share Aria's experiences alongside those of other youth who died by suicide, experienced suicidal ideation, or attempted suicide. We also attend to the experiences of the parents and mental health workers at the school, in pediatricians' offices, and in clinics around the community, all trying to keep kids safe and mourning when they cannot. Because we were already well known in Poplar Grove by the time of Aria's death (though we did not know her or her family beforehand), we, too, participated in the community response; Anna flew to Poplar Grove quickly to co-host, with a local clinical psychologist, a question-and-answer session on suicide prevention for the reeling Poplar Grove parents.

When faced with a death by suicide, *Why?* is in some ways an inherently unanswerable question. Suicide results from a constellation of risk factors and protective factors, from a person who can no longer answer our questions having exceeded some unknowable threshold of pain. Even in the rare cases when we have a note or journal,[2] we know the author was not in an ideal place to reflect or reason. Suicidal individuals are not irrational or unable to know their own minds, but testimonies like Aria's must be read as records of a particular moment and a particular mindset. Cultural factors make things trickier: most people are uncomfortable with death, and many of us have assumptions or biases attached to suicide. Over the centuries, this act has been variously understood as a sign of mental illness or pathology, a crime, and a sin. Suicide is stigmatized as unimaginable: each death is its own mystery, and the search for someone to blame all too easily creeps into conversation and gossip. Yet to identify the ways we can make the world worth living in for all youth—regardless of their diagnoses, experiences, resources, or psychological pain—we must extend a radical empathy, setting aside judgments about suicide and suicidal ideation as bad, wrong, or unspeakable, so that we can understand the experience from their point of view.

The way we, as social scientists, approach the question *Why?* in this case is through a research method called a social autopsy.[3,4] Social autopsies are a way to help uncover the root causes of a surprising or disproportionately high rate of a particular cause of death, centered on a geographic location. This involves gathering testimonies about a person's life and the circumstances surrounding their death, then considering a number of accounts in aggregate. The method is not perfect, particularly in the case of suicide: grieving loved ones can have biased perceptions of the decedent's motives, even very close connections may not have known what was going on, and some are understandably limited if they do not wish or have the capacity to share their experiences. To account for some of these limitations, we also work to triangulate information, check facts, and speak to as many people as possible.

The results of the social autopsies we conducted in Poplar Grove revealed two patterns that hint at how this specific place generates disproportionate rates of psychological pain and exacerbates vulnerability to suicide. By digging into the first—the distinct way that youth here spoke about the pressure to "measure up" as a "good" kid from a "good" family and the shameful feelings they attached to their perceptions that they had failed to meet expectations—we see in this chapter how the community's social environment fomented adolescents' psychological pain. In turn, in Chapter 4, we will see how shame got in the way of seeking and effectively getting help. Without disrupting these patterns, it will remain crushingly difficult to effectively prevent suicide in Poplar Grove.

3.1 THE PAIN OF NOT MEASURING UP

With her lively personality and theater experience, it made sense that Madison broke the ice in one of our earliest youth focus groups, responding first to our typical opening question: "What's it like to grow up in Poplar Grove?"

"It can be pretty stressful," Madison admitted. "A lot of people around you might have *more*." Though she got great grades and never got in trouble (more precisely, she never got caught), Madison lived in what she and others described as the poor side of town. "There's not a lot of money in my house," the teen confessed. "My parents are constantly arguing about money situations." Quickly, Madison noted that her parents were "good at school," and so it was hard to tell what happened, why their educational accomplishments had left them still worrying about money in adulthood.

Over time, we would learn that much of Madison's stress centered around her project to "make it" in Poplar Grove—to succeed, make her parents proud, and secure her route to a prosperous adulthood (all without financially burdening her family). In Chapter 2, Madison was among the teens who thought the mental health problems plaguing their peers stemmed from the community's high-pressure atmosphere. She explained, "Some people are just like so stressed out, like they can't [handle it]." Madison continued:

> Like, they have so many expectations put on to them. Like, their parents are like, "Oh. You're going to get into school for sports. You're going to have like a 4.5 GPA," which is like practically impossible. "You're going to do all this stuff. You're going to be like top of your class." And it's just like, they can't deal with the stress because they don't . . . They weren't like that, in like, elementary school and middle school. Like, they weren't pressured, but now that it's like junior year of high school, going to college: "This is your future, and I'm planning your future out for you. So, you have to do good so you can live up to my dreams and not yours." And so that's what happens a lot. . . . And then, sometimes people just, they just can't live with anything anymore.

Despite her use of the third person, Madison was voicing her own experience. The weight of her parents' expectations, if not the weight of the world, seemed heavy on her shoulders. She cared deeply, and the stress intensified as she increased her load of Advanced Placement (AP) classes. Her vision of her adulthood depended on getting excellent grades she might parlay into a scholarship. As she explained, it would need to be enough to carry her through graduate school; otherwise, the consequences could be dire:

> I need to pick my grades up, because I'm not going to get into a good college just to go and major into Veterinary Sciences . . . 'cause I'm going to go to college for like, 10 years [including vet school], and I'm not going to make the money and I'm going to have thousands and thousands of dollars of college loans. So, if I don't pick my game up, I'm not going to succeed in life. And I'm going to be stuck doing a job that I don't want to do, seven days a week, all the time, and I'm going to hate it.

To Madison, like many other Poplar Grove youth, adults could turn out either successful or miserable. You made it—or you hated your life. The pressure she felt from her parents was, in that sense, understandable:

> I would always have all this pressure on me to do everything that [my parents] wanted me to, and then it kind of grew into the fact that I really couldn't do what they wanted me to, to the best of my ability because I had so much going on. And they don't believe me a lot when I'm like, "I need to stay home because I don't feel good." Like, I did that the other day and my mom's like, "School comes first. You're not going to get into vet school with Cs."

Flatly, Madison recalled her retort: "I'm not going to get into vet school if I'm dead."

Conflict was normal between Madison and her parents. "I mean, my dad thinks it's a joke that I cut myself," Madison shared. "My mom doesn't understand it either," she said as she started to cry. "It's like parents *don't care!* And that's the problem."[ii] Of course, Madison's parents *do* care. In fact, Madison made it a point to tell us how her mother prioritized mental health, speaking of their home as a safe space for any friends experiencing mental health troubles and letting Madison use her phone at the dinner table if she was chatting with a friend in emotional distress. "She's kind of like [my friends'] second mom." Madison's parents didn't understand her self-harm, nor why kids couldn't just "get" the grades or keep going after losing a close friend to suicide in middle school, yet they cared. They got Madison into therapy when she needed it. But it seemed as though Madison's childhood was so different from her parents' that there was a divide between them. The inability of Madison's parents to fully understand or know how to deal with all their daughter had been through harmed Madison's sense of support and love.

Madison's story was also full of comparisons. Other parents, she thought, were able to serve as lifeguards for their kids, but Madison saw the academic opportunities her parents' sacrifices afforded her as being thrown in the academic deep end. Her parents didn't have the personal experience to help her navigate the intense stressors of Poplar Grove High School (PGHS) or the finances to get her the kinds of extra training or tutoring other Poplar Grove families used to ensure their kids' success. Not having access to these extra resources was quite salient in Madison's account, in fact. She suspected that she would lose her mind from stress or sleep deprivation, trying to keep up with peers who could afford access to private tutors, private coaches, private voice lessons. Motivation was not a problem: one got the sense that if someone would just tell Madison *how* to succeed, she'd gladly hop to it. And yet Madison felt like none of the adults in her life got it. They couldn't help her find balance or how to make it with her limited resources, so they just doubled down on the pressure.

Sociologists call Madison's tendency to look around and notice others' assets and accomplishments social comparison. It is a fairly universal human behavior that helps us form relationships, because watching others helps us understand how members of one group or another "should" behave and assess how our own actions measure up to those group expectations.[5] In other words, social comparison is how we figure out what is expected of us, whether we fit in or belong, and whether we are meeting the expectations of our salient social groups (and, thus, avoid being ostracized). Most individuals, like Madison, seek out group members they see as "better" than themselves in a variation called upward social comparison. Again, this practice is not inherently damaging. Upward social comparisons can encourage self-enhancement and self-improvement. They can inspire us to see what is possible. But it's not tough to see how they could be problematic. Madison, for instance, often used comparisons with friends and peers to discuss her inability to fulfill school and community expectations; this comparison process was painful and denigrating as opposed to informative and inspirational. These exchanges also revealed how central "making it" in Poplar Grove was to Madison's happiness and well-being. Peers who were making it, she figured, had little reason to feel bad like she did. "Like, my friend Kimberly is really good at volleyball, and her team has won lots of competitions. *And so whenever she's sad, I'm like, 'Dude, you're like the reason your volleyball team wins!'* " [emphasis added] Madison continued, using an anecdote about her friend Marika, who, we knew, had serious self-harm and psychological issues:

MADISON: And then, my other friends are really good singers . . . like, my friend Marika, she's like, "Yeah, my vocal teacher said . . . She's chosen me as one of her two students that she [thinks] could . . . audition for a choir at Carnegie Hall." . . . And I'm like, "Dude, that's great. *And you doubt yourself so much. Yet, here you are having this great opportunity put before you that not a lot of people have.*" And then a lot of my friends are really good at their sports, and I'm like, "Dude, you have like full-ride scholarships coming next year. Like, I can tell. Like, you have great grades. You have great looks. You have great friends. You have great sports. You have great family. Like, so you have like this whole thing like set up! You're going to get like a full-ride scholarship . . . [and] go to whatever college you want to." So, it's like a lot of my friends do a lot of stuff. And I'm just kind of like, "I do stuff sometimes." [emphasis added]

ANNA: What stuff do you do?

MADISON: I mean, I dance. I sing. But I don't really like see myself as good at any of it. Like, there's always someone better at it than me, usually. Most of the time.

The message that anyone who was demonstrably "making it"—who had auditions in New York City or athletic championships to their credit—couldn't or shouldn't legitimately have mental health problems was, incidentally, a widespread belief in Poplar Grove. It made everything seem more agonizing for Madison, whose perception that she constantly failed to live up to the full vision of an ideal Poplar Grove youth eroded her resilience. She was grieving, sleep deprived, and overscheduled. Add the stress of narrow expectations and the incessant social comparisons, and Madison's life felt miserably painful. "There's like a lot of people who are like, 'Oh, it gets so much better after high school.' Like, 'It gets so much better after middle school. It'll be fine tomorrow,'" Madison recounted. But Madison was getting pretty damn tired of being told to wait 'til tomorrow to feel *fine*.

Madison attempted suicide, both before we met her and in the time since. Thankfully, she survived. She knew suicide wasn't her only option—she dreamed of other ways to leave Poplar Grove behind—and she understood the devastation suicide brought to friends and family. Mark, her middle school best friend, had died by suicide, after all. But that intimate relationship had also shown her that suicide *was* an option. "He was the only person that understood me," Madison explained, "and like talked to me, and like helped me out with my problems." She continued:

Mark had so many issues of his own, and now he doesn't have them anymore. Like, how great would that be? To not have to like go through your life thinking about every little thing that you do . . . Like, "Oh, crap. I just like looked down when that person was looking at me. Are they going to think I'm a freak or something?" Like, you know? So, it's just kind of like, "What a great idea." Like, you don't have to like deal with any of your problems anymore. Like, you could just be.

In larger, more diverse places, teens might be able to identify and "try on" many different ways to "be a teen." The adolescent period of developmental identity instability in such places offers more varied examples of "making it." Poplar Grove was absent this minor luxury. Madison was not alone in feeling squeezed out of her small town's narrow, one-size-fits-all mold, nor in feeling this made it too difficult to live a life worth living. Many of her peers noted difficulties ranging from suicidal thoughts to "just" anxiety, depression, or self-harm. The benefits of smaller communities, idealized by fiction and punditry,[6] in many ways come with real downsides. Not all people from the same place have the same skills, capacities, resources, or desires to fulfill a set of narrow expectations, to follow a single route to performing a particular, incredibly important role-identity. What's more, structural factors constrain the attainability of certain honors—only one kid can be the lead in the school play or quarterback on the varsity football team—but where being less than perfect is the same as failure, then "failure" is inherent in the youth status system. Singular identities may offer a certain clarity, predictability, and stability, but threats to them— for example, failing to meet expectations and being punished by self or others—are extraordinarily painful.[7] In part, this is because the loss of the right to play that role is synonymous with not belonging to the only group that matters to a person, to their community.

3.2 STANDING OUT IN LIFE AND DEATH

As we collected testimonies about Quinn Davis from her friends and family, it became clear that she, too, had suffered the pain of being different in Poplar Grove. She had hidden this pain well, publicly embracing herself as someone who stood out from the crowd. Vivacious with an "infectious personality," Quinn was very much admired. Universally, people described her as a "wild," "hair on fire" kind of girl. They told us she loved to pull stunts. One time, when her family insisted she go to the fancy private school a few blocks from PGHS, she ditched school to sneak into a friend's math class at PGHS. She took a seat . . . to the shock of the teacher and the baffled delight of her friend. "Do you even go to this school?" the teacher asked. Quinn laughed and ran out of the room, her friend recounted with a giggle.

Quinn's antics featured in many of our interviews. When she ran for class president, we heard, her campaign slogan was "Flavas for Davis," and she walked around school handing out donuts as a vote-getting stunt. When she was chosen to give morning announcements on the public address system, she screamed into the microphone, rousing her sleepy classmates with a 7 a.m. "GOOOOOD MORNING POPLAR GROVE!!!" And on school-spirit days, Quinn always went overboard. For Homecoming, Quinn colored her skin red (PGHS's color) with magic markers, just to make sure she was the most spirited person in the room.

Without a doubt, this girl danced to her own tune. Victoria, a close family friend, told us she had known Quinn since she was a toddler: "I just saw [a girl who declared] 'I am my own person, and you're not going to put me in a box.'" Sometimes people thought of Quinn, who proudly parked her funky classic car among the crowd of BMWs and Lexuses outside PGHS, as "eccentric," though the ones who were close to her treasured Quinn as beautifully unique. Leah, one of Quinn's closest and oldest friends, said through tears:

Quinn . . . taught me that it's okay to be the person you are. . . . It doesn't matter what other people think at all. She taught me that, and I don't know, I've always been kind of, like, weird, I guess. [Laughter] But she kind of made me embrace that because I realize that some-body could love me for who I was anyways. So, she was kinda the first person to show me that.

For this alone, Leah will always treasure Quinn's friendship. Leah continued:

With her being gone, the thing that I carry with me is I know she would not want me to conform to other people's expectations or what other people want for me. She made me know that I can feel free to be who I am.

That role modeling has extended outward so that Leah and her best friend Kaitlyn both credit Quinn—and losing Quinn—as transformational. She emboldened them to become brave cultural rebels who sometimes hang out with their parents, going to "dad music shows" just because they actually like to (even if it's not "cool").

At the same time, insights from Quinn's friends and family attest that her uniqueness came at a cost. Quinn wanted to be accepted. She bought into Poplar Grove's esprit de corps and insisted her parents let her go to PGHS rather than the private high school nearby. And at PGHS, she was highly involved: she ran for class president, excelled in all the right AP classes, and lent her voice to the school in those morning announcements. Everyone knew her and her family—Quinn's classmates called them "legendary" and were in awe of their cool musical tastes (*not* your typical "dad" music) and fabulous vacations. Quinn even had her own boat—perhaps, in this waterfront community, not incredibly attention-grabbing, but still very cool.

And yet Quinn hadn't always had an easy time maintaining friendships, a critical source of social support in adolescence. An old childhood friend named Danica told us she had drifted away from Quinn because she could be overly possessive: "[Quinn would] get really frustrated with the fact that I had other really close friends. . . . And I remember at [a] birthday party, too, we watched some Lindsay Lohan movie, and there was a chair, and she made sure that she sat in the chair with me, and nobody else sat in the chair with me, and it was just the two of us." Danica felt so smothered that she not only ended her friendship with Quinn, but encouraged other kids to stay away from her, too. The guilt still stuck with Danica. "I had moved into this new group of friends," Danica explained, "and I loved them, they were my best friends." She continued:

We all played sports together, we liked all the same boys, and we were kind of in that in-group of girls. And then they met Quinn in one of their classes, and I remember being really frustrated, 'cause they were kind of like *my* friends, *my* new friends. . . . And then they were all friends with her, but I didn't like her anymore. . . . And [sighs] it's definitely one of the worst things I did, like, "I don't like her, she's not cool, blah blah blah." And they were all still friends with her, they didn't listen to me, which was fine. But then after a couple months, she does get really overbearing, and she does get kind of in your face and stuff. And then they're all, like, "You know what, Danica, you're right, she's not cool, blah blah blah. . . ."

I still feel bad about it, and at the time I felt bad about it, 'cause I'm, like, [its] definitely one of the shittiest things I've ever done . . . she ended up finding people. I'd feel worse if she never ended up finding people. But even then, I think there's just, like, flitting through and seeing where she did fit in, 'cause she was so different from most people.

Small conflicts like these are normal (friendships can be quite unstable in the preteen and teenage years), but the importance of friends and feeling accepted by peers during adolescence cannot be overstated. Teens, especially those struggling with psychological challenges, can be protected profoundly through the loyalty of just one or two close friends. The story Danica told took place years before Quinn's death, though it demonstrates some of the ferocity of young people's bonds. It also shows that, even for someone with the sort of audacious coolness others described in Quinn, being "so different from most people" can be painful.

Leah, however, recognized that her friend's apparent immunity to conformist pressures wasn't the whole story. Quinn "cared what people thought," she said, and continued:

But she didn't let them know that. She actually cared, like, a lot, but she was just a little crazy, so she just did stuff anyways. [Laughs] And so people kind of always recognized her as that. Especially in high school, she started doing her own thing 'cause we had our own group of friends, and she wasn't spending time with people that she didn't feel like she belonged with, like really sporty, athletic types. Like, she realized that wasn't her, and so she kind of was finding herself a little more too. I don't think she realized that, though. She always felt really really lost. . . . She tried so hard to make everybody like her, and it worked. Like, most everybody loved her.

For her part, Leah remembered that Quinn "wore herself ragged trying to please everybody and trying to do the things that she thought she had to do," to "kind of just be what everybody wanted." Quinn's older sibling fit the mold in Poplar Grove pretty well. It appears Quinn wished, at least to some degree, that she did, too.

Quinn left behind a brief suicide note, which caused her mother Cora to dig through her room and dissect her diary. In her diary, Cora found a table that lists of pros and cons of suicide from an entry a few days before she ended her life (see Table 3.1).[iii] A number of the entries are oriented toward what others think or feel about her. Her indication that she might escape the "bitches," "haters," and people "getting mad at [her]" can be read as a deep desire to escape others' judgments.

Quinn's table also hints at the psychological strain of the academic and social pressures of Poplar Grove. Notably, at the top of her list of suicide's "pros" are "no school," "no college," and "no more stress." Later on in her diary, in the entry for what Quinn described as her "last day of

Table 3.1 TABLE FROM QUINN'S DIARY

Suicide

Pros	Cons
No school	Secrets coming out
No work	Guilt
No college	Ruining everyones lives
No more stress	Family losing money
No more bitches	Rumors would fly about me
No one getting mad at me	
No more haters	

school . . . forever," she mused on the possibility of getting help instead of ending her life. That, however, would mean still dealing with school and the pressure to not let people down. She wrote:

> Everyone would be balls happy if I stayed alive but then I have to live with the consequences; missing school, makeup work, stuck in a mental hospital, medicated. And then there's the things that would never change. I would still have to go to college, work and worry about money, continue to be yelled at and letting down everyone.

Recall, that in Chapter 2, Kaitlyn shared that this pressure that Quinn felt—that everyone feels—was the most salient thing for us, as researchers, to understand about growing up in Poplar Grove:

> Honestly, I just say the most emphasis should be put on the pressure that people feel around here. And even when I try to explain it to my parents, it's hard for them to understand, and it's really hard to explain. . . . They don't realize how much pressure we put on ourselves as young adults. Some people don't pressure themselves but when kids do, they can be really hard on themselves, especially when they've been kind of raised thinking that they're not good enough.

It's "not on purpose," Kaitlyn added, "but that's just kind of how it ends up a lot of the time."

Quinn and Madison's stories share a startling similarity: the pain that can result from struggling to meet community expectations and ideals. Whether girls who felt they didn't have what it takes (be it money, talent, or some intangible source of merit), like Madison, or popular, "ideal-typical"[iv] young women, like Quinn (or Carrie who we met in Chapter 2), who seemingly had it all, we repeatedly heard the corrosive pain that came with adolescent girls thinking they did not measure up. (And as we will see in Section 3.4, this pain was echoed, though not as loudly, among the boys.)

3.3 WHEN "PERFECT" IS NOT ENOUGH

Michelle was a truly ideal-typical Poplar Grove youth. She was good at sports and school, and her peers remembered her as a warm, loving friend. "There was something about her," Molly said fondly, recalling that, like Quinn, Michelle played harmless jokes: "She would always steal your keys . . . go into my car and drive it and park it down the road." Krista, who was a junior when she met Michelle, who was then a freshman, spoke of the teen's magnetism: "I thought she was really cool and I wanted to be her friend, I feel, like, she's that type of person where, like, I just wanted to be her friend because she was so cool." We heard her described as attractive, gregarious, sarcastic, "a special person [with] really good energy," and, in Beth's admiring words, "unapologetically herself." Moments later, Beth paused to add, "it's weird because she had [those qualities], but at the same time it felt like there was also something dark there."

On the outside, her friends confided as our conversation continued, Michelle *seemed* a perfect Poplar Grove teen, a popular, pretty, high achiever who made it all look easy. Yet those closest to her knew she was "self-conscious" and concerned about what others thought. "Michelle was very into her image because, she was always, she had the best outfits on," Vanessa commented, "I think [it was a] 'looking good made her feel good' kinda thing. But, she was definitely always put together. You could never see her in sweatpants unless she was out on the soccer field." Michelle had been hospitalized a few times for treatment related to depression and an eating disorder—problems her friends attributed to her being under pressure. Even so, it was a real surprise to classmates when Michelle died by suicide:

BECCA: Yeah. Michelle was a star.
MADISON: She had like the best grades.
BECCA: Yeah, the best grades. She was always president. Yeah, like Michelle was the most everything that anybody could ever want to be. She was beautiful, tall, blond.

MADISON: She was great at sports. She was really thin.

BECCA: Exactly and everyone loved her and then one day you walked into school and saw everyone crying and it's like what's happening? You walk into your first period teacher and she says well, Michelle is dead.

MADISON: And I'm like what? I did not see that coming. Like really no one saw it coming at all.

BECCA: No one ever. At all. Then you're thinking. Oh, well there are these people who may be contemplating it, then there are these people you know for sure, because you've seen them in that slump and have seen their Facebook statuses about it like, "Oh life is so horrible. Why do people do these things?" It's just weird to think about how many people could be thinking about suicide and killing themselves and stuff.

Michelle's best friend Molly confided, "The way I've always thought about it is that she wanted to be perfect and needed to see herself as perfect, but didn't and couldn't, and no one could convince her that she was perfect except herself. She couldn't do that." Molly continued:

I feel like she never felt like she could be perfect in her own eyes, and she had explained this to me just a week and a half before she died. She was telling me, "No matter how many people tell me that I'm skinny or pretty or whatever, it doesn't matter because it matters what I think." I feel like she didn't think that things were going to get better and that she was ever going to be happy with herself. Even though on the outside it's like super athletic, varsity athlete, stellar grades, headed for a great college to play lacrosse, that is what it looks like from the outside, and pretty and skinny and all of those things, but to her, she wasn't who she wanted to be. I guess with her personality, she felt like she wasn't doing everything right, and she told me all these things, and obviously, I tried to talk to her about it, but I didn't know how serious that really was. That was the end of October, so obviously that was not very long before.

Michelle, we learned, differed from Aria in that her family emphasized their expectation that she would live up to—live out—Poplar Grove's ideals. Vanessa went so far as to say:

I think her parents had a lot to do with [Michelle's low self-esteem], which is awful. Not so much her dad. I would say her mom, who has definitely loosened up since then, but I always played sports with [Michelle's sister] Everly and Michelle, and her mom was always the one that was just like, "You can do more," pushing them further and further. So I think it was just the pressure from her mom. And I think [having a successful sister] was also very hard on her because they both excelled at everything, so it was definitely a race between the two of them. So it was pressure from each other, from the mom on themselves. I think she just couldn't handle all of those voices telling her what to do.

Other friends pointed to the larger sources of pressure they all faced in Poplar Grove. Krista wondered whether "it had to do with the culture, like suburban culture" of the town, in which all of the girls agreed socialization meant internalizing incredibly high measures of success. To Beth, Michelle's struggle was "understandable, when you are . . . constantly surrounded by people who are achieving certain things that you feel like you have to be like them." In another moment, Beth summarized the culture by saying failure was "not an option" for Poplar Grove youth. The world these teens inhabited presented a difficult set of requirements. They had to do well—really spectacularly well—but also, according to Beth, talk as though their successes were not enough, "like they weren't satisfied with it." It had become the norm for high achievers to be "put on blast" by "individuals and organizations," according to Beth. Those high achievers "want people to know their achievements and stuff 'cause they thought it was *cool*." She continued that high achievers "talk about their achievement, but [act] disappointed . . . in their achievements so that other people go, 'Wow, I can't even get to your level, but you're not satisfied with that level, so I must be doing terribly with my life.' So, I think that's something that happened a lot."

That must have been hard to hear for kids who were struggling to get by, more so because so many of the youth who died by suicide had been among those high achievers—the kids who embodied Poplar Grove's ideals. Krista said her friend Michelle had been "trying to find worth in things that she felt, like, she could *never do perfectly*." Poignantly, she concluded, "I guess she felt like there was no reason to keep living, because nothing was giving her the worth that she wanted." Perfectionism in a tight-knit community where everybody knows your business, the ideal youth is visible and known, and yet the standards of perfection are a moving target, is a dangerous cultural directive: anything short of an always-out-of-reach "perfect" may feel like a shameful failure.

3.4 THE PAIN OF FAILURE

Thus far, we have looked at the stories of young women who struggled with the painful mismatch between *who they thought they were* and *who they thought they should be*. We also found, more prevalent among the young men we got to know through interviews with families and friends, that youth suicides coincided with instances in which youth had more concrete evidence of their "failure," such as tangles with the law. Young men, however, were not immune to the agony of measuring themselves against perfection and believing they came up short. Meet Brian.

Brian was dreamy. Handsome. Artistic. Smart. Sociable. "He was really cool," shared his friend Chloe. "Kind of introverted. Super-hot, you know? Blond hair, blue eyes, really artsy. . . . And he was a really nice sensitive sweet guy." Brian's father Bruce made less of the young man's looks, perhaps, but said much the same: "He always had girlfriends and he was pretty sensitive with those relationships . . . he took things to heart and—but he was also happy-go-lucky, damn the torpedoes, did stuff he shouldn't do, [tried to] get away with it." Bruce laughed, maybe remembering some specific instance as he added, "He always got caught." At another point, Bruce said, "If he wanted to do something, he'd do it. I'm sure he partied. I'm sure he got into all kinds of things he shouldn't have. But he was a responsible, sensitive kid, and—when he wanted to be—intelligent, getting an A in some subjects that I wouldn't get an A in."

When Brian went off to a well-ranked state university, Bruce was incredibly proud. It was exactly what Bruce and his wife Rose wanted for their children. And so when they lost Brian to suicide, they just couldn't wrap their minds around it. Like so many parents, they were searching for the answer to a very big question: What happened to make their child feel life was unlivable?

Father and son, Bruce and Brian led very different lives, just as Bruce intended. "I grew up in a small, rural town in Wisconsin and . . . we lived in a small town and went to small schools. We had what we needed, but we didn't have any extra luxuries," Bruce explained. When it came to their own family, Bruce and Rose were "trying to give these kids all they—all we think they need. And they're smart kids, they're all in college, they're all straight-As. I mean, what is it? What's the problem?"

It's hard for parents to see the harm in pushing children to fit into a particular mold, especially when it is so normalized. Getting good grades, doing well in college, these feel necessary to the kind of future that Bruce imagined for his son. It was inconceivable to Bruce that, when Brian went off to college, he got an F in psychology—his major—but aced other, seemingly harder courses like statistics. Bruce, a self-employed entrepreneur, knew he could be demanding with the kids: "I'm a driver," he told Anna, "and I would drive the kids to be productive citizens in society." So, too, could their extended family, who lived in Poplar Grove and were highly "involved." By way of example, Bruce offered: "I'm sure my, my mother-in-law [will question the kids] like, 'So what are you doing about this, and what are you doing about that?'" Theirs is a family that values having a plan and taking action.

Comparing his three children, Bruce sighed that Brian was "a follower, not a leader." The "other two are more leaders. Marianne wants to be in charge of everything—and she is—and Cheryl knows what she's doing and she's got her little plan planned out, and you don't know what that plan is, but she does." Bruce thought that Brian, on the other hand, spent too much time following peers who didn't value hard work and family the way his parents did. "We talked about that from time to time, you know," the father recalled of sit-downs with Rose and Brian. Bruce continued:

> [We'd say,] "You need to be a leader, not a follower. You are following these guys down these bad paths." . . . And he'll go, "I know you're frustrated, Mom, that you don't think I'm doing the right stuff, but I know exactly what I'm doing." So, he's kinda like that. But so that's the—that's really the story. . . . His friends, he'd do stuff like he'd be [caught with an] open container [of alcohol] at college and get in a fight and come home with black eyes and shave his head, and all these extreme[s].

Tellingly, Bruce mentioned that others, outside the family, commented on the many ways Brian seemed to be straying from community norms: "And this is a very conservative, loving family I'm talking about, and he comes home with his head shaved. Everyone's like, 'What is going on, Bruce, with your kid?!'"

In some ways, Brian's story is similar to what we heard about Quinn, Michelle, and so many of the other Poplar Grove youth who attempted or died by suicide. According to his friends and family, Brian struggled with depression, at least partially tied to the fact he felt that he failed to measure up to his family and community's expectations. "I think with Brian, a huge struggle for him was to fit in," explained his friend Avery, "because he was—I mean, he was like laid-back, a jokester, like he wasn't really preppy or anything. And, I think he felt a lot of pressure to be like 'I have to find a sport I'm good at. I have to do this. I had to make everybody happy.'" The difference was that, unlike most of the young women who died by suicide in Poplar Grove, Brian had managed to cope, graduate high school, and go to college before circumstances overwhelmed his efforts.

People back home in Poplar Grove were aware of many of Brian's troubles at college—and the judgments were harsh. His girlfriend weathered peers' derision as they talked about Brian as a loser who flunked out. He didn't, actually—he got kicked out of the dorms for smoking pot, and so he was forced to move back into his parents' house and commute to his university classes. He also got into legal trouble (perhaps pot, perhaps for some other minor infraction—Bruce said he really couldn't remember) that landed him in front of a judge. The judge laid it out for him: "Your dad can't help you anymore. You're the guy. You're it. Stay out of the court system."

Unfortunately, for whatever reason, Brian couldn't. The night before his death was spent in jail. When his parents arrived to post bail, their son was devastated. Bruce "wasn't real happy," either, he remembered, but he was determined to find lawyers, to figure out how to prevent Brian from losing his driver's license and his vehicle. Brian tried to tell him not to bother. In hindsight, Bruce regretted brushing that comment off. As Brian insisted "Well, I'm not gonna be here for this. I'm not gonna be here for that," Bruce just responded, "Of course you're going to be there." It didn't click until Bruce dropped by Brian's work to check in the day after his arrest and learned his son hadn't shown up. He remembered telling another employee, "This is something that could really be traumatic enough for him to do something terrible." He remembered the employee asking, "What are you talking about?" He remembered saying only one more word: "Suicide."

Coming home to find his son dead was like being in a movie, Bruce explained. Brian was already gone. The meaning had clicked too late.

Years later, Bruce still quietly questioned what had gone wrong. "I feel bad sometimes," Bruce admitted, "that maybe I drove him too hard." In his words, we could hear him grappling with what-ifs:

> I would be disappointed in Brian. . . . Did he hear me say that? Did I ever say, "I'm disappointed in Brian"? I didn't say that, but he shouldn't—he shouldn't be doing this stuff . . . I was harder on [Brian] than [Rose]—she's more of a pacifist and a "let's make his bed [for him]" . . . and I would be more like "let's *teach him* to make his own bed." I'm using an analogy, but that's kind of the way everything went with him.

Parents aren't perfect. And sometimes, sadly, they don't know what their children are going through or need from them until it's too late. Today, Bruce channels his sorrow, disappointment, and resignation—all the huge, unending feelings tied to his loss—into his surviving children, his life partner Rose, and his suicide prevention efforts. He has become a trusted adult for his children's friends, frankly talking to teens about mental health and lending a hand with the community's suicide prevention activities. He is willing to be honest and open, and is laying bare his own limitations, regrets, sorrows, and joys, in his interview with us and beyond, all in the hope that someone will finally figure out the big question: What are we doing wrong?

3.5 SIMILARITIES AND DIFFERENCES

Having gathered all of these accounts, the next step in our examination of youth suicide in Poplar Grove was to step back from the details and look for patterns. Pressure to succeed, which can be positive, fostered shame when these young people failed to meet community and family standards. There were, however, differences across the cases. Most uniquely, the young White women who died by suicide were generally still in high school, while young White men, like Brian, more often died shortly after graduating from high school. Further, young men's problems tended to hit a tipping point after they had contact with state institutions, particularly law enforcement and judges; to our knowledge, none of the young women who died had any prior institutional contacts other than psychiatric hospitals.

It is also worth noting variation in the teens' proximity to the sources of perfectionist pressures in their lives. Diffuse community expectations were felt keenly, yet home and family could provide a powerful place of refuge, as we saw with the cultural rebels in Chapter 2. When the cultural ideals were, instead, a constant refrain at home, it could amplify young people's sense of failure. Interviewees spoke about pushy parents as part of the reasons why Kennedy, Michelle, Brian, and other youth died, like

Julia's stories. Denise, whose close friend Julia died by suicide, for instance, felt Julia's parents were "all about keeping up appearances . . . you could be a hot mess in the comfort of your own home, but man, when you go out in public, you have to project this image of perfection." Parents need not be outwardly high-pressure—Aria's parents, for example, came across as fairly laid back, but they were also impressively creative, entrepreneurial, professional successes. We also learned that young people's striving was amplified by siblings, particularly siblings seen as living up to Poplar Grove's ideal in ways that might highlight their perceived shortcomings. For Julia, having an "absolutely stunning" sister who "did everything right" must have felt like having a live-in yardstick. The same can be said of Quinn's and Michelle's siblings, who similarly embodied cultural expectations and, by being so close, made those expectations real, concrete, and fundamentally important to youth. By the same token, having a less than ideal-typical family member could amplify pressure, as we saw with Madison, who was positioned as the "golden child" against the cautionary tale of her brother, who dropped out of high school, shocking their family. Perhaps she felt she was her parents' last chance to fulfill the Poplar Grove dream.

3.6 CONCLUSION

Again, while complexity goes hand in hand with suicide, if we step back, two clear patterns reveal the social roots of suicide. Severe psychological pain, whether stemming from a clinically diagnosable disorder or evidenced in behavioral expressions like self-harming, is a frequent feature in the psychological and emotional profiles of youth who die by suicide, in and beyond Poplar Grove. The second thread that winds through the stories of suicide in this community is the devastation of not meeting expectations. For many, Poplar Grove seemed to create and/or exacerbate psychological pain. The diffuse set of cultural expectations that make the town so desirable were reinforced at home, at school, among siblings and friends, with varying intensity and intentionality. Each group and setting had its own potential to amplify young people's sense of failure, to foster shame. Without oversimplifying suicide or attempting to downplay its devastating, cascading effects, suicide is a social phenomenon. We can look at these lost youth and imagine how intervening in the social environment could have eased the impact of "failures," or could have helped make young lives, always fraught, feel nonetheless livable.

Sociology has always held foundational insights about how people live together. One is that the cultural worlds we inhabit guide our behavior. Unlike a tattered old Rand McNally atlas stuffed under a car seat, however, these cultural road maps are endorsed and legitimated by the groups to which we belong, internalized and taken for granted by the group's members, and enforced via social sanctions should those members stray. Collectives like Poplar Grove, PGHS, or individual cliques within PGHS, however unintentionally, have the authority, for instance, to shun—and for most humans, a loss of social belonging (real or imagined) is the ultimate threat. Equally powerful for ensuring adherence to the cultural roadmaps is self-regulation—the act of policing oneself. Because enforcement of a person's behavior by other group members—via shunning or the gossip we discussed in earlier chapters—takes time and energy, groups usually also try to get members to self-regulate by internalizing group values. Self-regulation means that group members often conform to group expectations even in private moments, when other group members aren't around or when other group members have no idea what they're thinking, feeling, or doing. To be clear, no matter how spectacularly an individual in Poplar Grove had messed up, no one—NO ONE—in this community would ever think suicide was a reasonable choice. Yet youth, who had been born and raised in this context, had internalized the message that messing up was absolutely unacceptable, even if no one found out. Often without giving their community, their family, or their friends a chance to change their minds, some youth came to see their lives as not worth living and took tragic action.

Both sources of social control—external and self-regulation—are plainly evident in Poplar Grove. The tight-knit nature of the community made it easy to monitor and punish youth and adults for the sake of course correction, while the coherent, narrow cultural ideals made it easy for youth and adults to know what they should be doing and avoid consequences by course-correcting themselves. Frequently, gossip was a tool of punishment carrying strong judgmental tones or even explicitly calling out community members for their role in youth suicides (whether in general or with regard to a specific death). Parents who lost their children to suicide often found themselves surrounded by a web of support—food arriving, funerals well attended, check-in calls from local faith leaders or neighbors—that also brought in close the judging "looks" of the community. Not meeting society's expectations came with social consequences, and so a narrow set of shared cultural beliefs generated pressure for youth, for families, and for schools and mental health workers. That pressure was a nuisance to some youth, adults, and families who decided when to follow and when to circumvent the basic rules of the game, knowing full well there could be consequences. For others, that specter magnified and multiplied the usual—or unusual—stressors of life and contributed to mental health issues.

The fear of failure figured heavily in what we found as a unifying explanation for why youth died by suicide in Poplar Grove. Kids in Poplar Grove who lived up to the community's intense expectations were pressured to keep it up or risk the social and psychological pain of failure. It means managing the *fear* of failure, which appeared to lurk around every corner—recall from Chapter 2 that superstar Shannon, taking over as team captain, feared she might ruin their rich legacy of state championships, while Madison catastrophized her grades and feared she would end working a crappy, seven-day-a-week job. Those who did fail, objectively or subjectively, who could not achieve at the highest school, sport, and social levels, grappled with managing the *shame* of failure. Shame, our most powerful social emotion, evolved as a sort of compass to help keep us on the right course in our collective's map. We may feel it around others, and others may even actively invoke shame, but its true strength derives from its ability to be triggered when we are alone. When we feel others believe that not our behavior, but our *self* is deficient, contemptible, corrupting, or polluting, we are feeling shame. It makes us want to hide, to tear our skin off, to do anything to manage the unbearable pain of shame.

Unfortunately, shame is very difficult to talk about, and most people attempt to manage it alone rather than sharing their pain with friends or family. When it is left untended, though, shame can become highly toxic. It can fuel intense anger that erupts outward, externalized onto the people seen as triggering the shame. Or it can intensify inward, in a painful cocktail of hard emotions that include grief, fear, and anger.[8] Shame is an emotion to take seriously for its role in psychological pain. And this socially induced pain is the exhausting burden carried by youth in Poplar Grove. The general prohibition against talking about shame mixed with the local expectations for perfection serve to dangerously stymie one of the healthiest protections against mental suffering and suicide: help-seeking. To seek help was to admit a sort of ultimate failure in Poplar Grove. And as we shall see in the next chapter, this shame plays a role in constraining the types of behaviors and effective policies that could actually prevent suicide.

NOTES

i. To allow Aria's full voice and as much of her experience to come through as possible, we have faithfully transcribed her handwritten words, leaving grammatical, spelling, and punctuation choices.

ii. We connected Madison to mental health care after this exchange, care that she stuck with for years.

iii. We share excerpts from Quinn's diary with explicit permission from her parents.

iv. "Ideal-typical" is a useful sociological descriptor that refers to a set of attributes that are "typically" considered "ideal" for a particular kind of person in a particular place or social group. It's meant to capture the standard for social comparison in a particular place.

REFERENCES

1. Joiner T. *Why People Die by Suicide*. Cambridge, MA: Harvard University Press; 2005.

2. Pestian J, Matykiewicz P, Linn-Gust M. What's in a Note: Construction of a Suicide Note Corpus. *Biomedical Informatics Insights*. 2012;5:1–6.

3. Scourfield J, Fincham B, Langer S, Shiner M. Sociological Autopsy: An Integrated Approach to the Study of Suicide in Men. *Social Science and Medicine*. 2012;74(4):466–473.

4. Timmermans S, Prickett PJ. The Social Autopsy. *Sociological Methods & Research*. 2021. doi: 10.1177/00491241211036163.

5. Buunk AP, Gibbons FX. Social Comparison: The End of a Theory and the Emergence of a Field. *Organizational Behavior and Human Decision Processes*. 2007;102(1):3–21.

6. Wuthnow R. *The Left Behind: Decline and Rage in Rural America*. Princeton, NJ: Princeton University Press; 2018.

7. Thoits PA. Multiple Identities and Psychological Well-Being: A Reformulation and Test of the Social Isolation Hypothesis. *American Sociological Review*. 1983;48(2):174–187.

8. Scheff T. Shame and Conformity: The Deference Emotion System. *American Sociological Review*. 1988;53(3):395–406.

4

THE STIGMA OF HELP-SEEKING

Jim loved raising his family within Poplar Grove's community of support. Yet Jim's family kept secrets. Jim confessed quietly:

> To be honest, we keep it quiet. There's a few people I told—a couple of people at work that I'm very friendly with. I was very upset at the time and it was really hard, but I didn't really talk about it. We still don't. I mean, people know about it and I mean, yeah, obviously people know about it, but we really don't talk about it.
>
> I'm not sure why we're embarrassed. It gets this stigma. And, it's just a very painful period. The thought of my son dying for one thing, it's—I was so scared that I was gonna lose him, I mean, in that time period, I was really, really scared, and then when we sent him away, I was, I mean, that summer, I literally cried like almost all summer. I mean . . . I was so depressed myself . . . but we didn't talk to, we never really sat down and talked to anybody about it.

What was "it"? "It" was his son Ian's struggles with mental health. Ian had severe mood swings, excessive drug use, and repeated attempts to die by suicide, all of which led to the teen having frequent contact with the police. Jim and his wife Ella knew they needed help. Ian's struggles were simply beyond their capacities. So they turned to counselors, psychiatrists, and hospitalizations; they involved social workers and reached out to their pastor. Ian cycled in and out of psychiatric hospitalizations, but each time, he was released back to his family home shockingly quickly. Eventually, the stress was too much for the family. They felt that Ian needed space from his bad influences—the friends who always seemed ready to get drunk or high. Space that the all-too-brief local hospitalizations repeatedly failed to provide.

First, Jim and Ella sent Ian to live with an aunt out of state, but when he returned, Ian fell right back in with the same kids and the same patterns. "He [was] just totally out of control," Jim recalled. "I don't feel safe, my wife doesn't feel safe. The house is all busted up. We don't know what's going on, [and] one of the things we got frustrated about was the fact that . . . there was no consistency. I couldn't seem to get him like consistent care . . . [so] every time I'm talking to [a doctor, it's] a totally new guy . . . and then they give me their spin on it."

When a social worker pushed the family to consider sending Ian to a residential treatment center, they found hope again. Ian could get more thorough and consistent care, maybe even sort his "behavioral problems" from his "psychological problems." Jim said:

> We did a lot of research and we found a place in Arizona. It was kind of drastic [sending Ian away for so long], but . . . it was really good. I always felt it was the right thing to do. I don't have any regrets doing it. It was very hard for us to send him away. But he got there, and he did very well there. He didn't have any episodes or anything. 'Cause he's normally a good kid, I mean, that's the thing, he's—you meet him and you're like—what's going on here?

Jim coached his son: "If anybody asks you, you don't have to tell them about the treatment part, just it's just a boarding school." And Jim was relieved that Ian "bought into that." Indeed, Ian graduated from high school while at the Arizona facility. Jim said, "I was pretty, very happy . . . He finished the program." It wasn't, however, the end of Ian's struggles.

Ian returned with prescribed medications for "bipolar disorder," though the residential treatment center told his parents they didn't want to give

Ian the "stamp" of a formal diagnosis. Jim tried to check in with Ian and his feelings, but both found it uncomfortable. Jim reflected:

> He doesn't talk about this very often. He's very—he doesn't talk about his [problems], but . . . I asked him . . . from time to time, I mean, we don't broach the subject a whole lot, trying to bring up the past, but I try to make sure, I said, "do you feel suicidal?" "No, I'm fine, dad." Ever since then, he's just kinda, "yeah, I'm fine, dad."

A little defensively, the father continued haltingly:

> I hate to say "no one's told me to talk about it," but when we—he's never really talked about it. When we talk to him, I just make sure he's okay. I mean, "how ya feeling?" You know, trying—my thing is trying to—or at least I think I'm, you know, they're just kinda going along with this or no one's given me any other suggestions, just "talk about the way forward." *Feeling all right?* What's gonna happen now?

Again, Jim captures all his son's troubles—the suicide attempts, mental illness, and drug use—in one little word: *it*. *It* hangs like a specter over their family life. *It* makes Jim frustrated and sad. *It* makes him feel let down by all the therapists and psychiatrists and mental health workers who he felt never took the time to help him understand *how* to support Ian.

In fact, instead of addressing stigmatizing beliefs about mental illness—beliefs that can amplify the stress any one of us feels in talking about a topic soaked in painful emotions like fear, shame, and despair—Jim's recollections revealed ways mental health workers reinforced rather than eased the stigma of Ian's mental illness. They reinforced the notion that what Jim, Ian, and the family were going through was something embarrassing, something stigmatizing. For example, the facility insisting that it avoided diagnoses that may "stamp" a child in some fundamental way amplified the sense that a diagnosis was not an informative label that could guide treatment, unlock medical resources, and facilitate communication with future psychiatrists or psychologists, but rather an undesirable and unshakeable negative mark.[1,2] It also may have made the mental illness seem less real, less like a medical condition that warrants treatment and more like something to get through privately.

No matter what he did to help his son—keep him home, send him away—Jim felt judged by the mental health specialists, like he "couldn't win." Jim confided:

> That was very disturbing. I was looking for somebody *to help me help him*, but I wasn't getting [that from clinicians]. I was getting, "what the heck did you do wrong? You did that, really? You shouldn't have been doing that" . . . maybe why the embarrassment came out and me and my wife talk a lot about it between us. I mean, we talk about that part of [our experience]. We'll be embarrassed or [feel like we] shouldn't tell people, but the thing we talk about is just trying to protect [Ian]. That stigma. That's the only thing I was really worried about, too, was the stigma I didn't want attached to [Ian].

For his part, Ian was no more eager to embrace a diagnosis. "I don't want to talk about the past," Ian told his father (who told us). He knew the stigma that would attach to him as soon as he told therapists his entire story, including the history of suicide attempts. Thus, Jim took on the task of those disclosures, making sure every new doctor or therapist understood the full scope of Ian's difficulties. Still, just between father and son, Jim said, "We've kinda not talked about the actual attempt since then. He's embarrassed about it . . . that's why I have to bring it up [with the doctors]."

What was behind this acute embarrassment, beyond the usual reticence to talk about our worst days and hardest experiences? In our data on the community's beliefs about mental health, we can see that the town's strong culture is, with regard to this issue, also a judgmental culture. Mental health challenges are frequently seen as shameful, used as fodder for local gossip, and taken as evidence of not meeting local expectations about "good" kids and "good" families. What is unique about Ian's experience is that his father, Jim, was more willing than many to admit painful truths—that he felt embarrassed by his son's mental illness—in the context of our confidential research interview. Jim was also persistent, committed, and thorough in his search for the best mental health help for his son. Despite negative experiences with help-seeking, Jim never gave up. He also had the money, thanks to his professional career, to pay for what Ian needed, no matter how threadbare insurance coverage could be for mental health treatment. But none of that was a foregone conclusion. It must have been really tough for Jim, his wife, and Ian to continue pushing forward and trying to pursue effective help. It took perseverance. And frankly, it was made far harder because, as we learned speaking with other families in Poplar Grove, the community simply wasn't open about the problems that came before the suicide deaths that haunted their American idyll. Some would only tell us about their children's struggles after we turned off our audio recorder and promised to keep their stories "off the record."

In Poplar Grove, mental health stigma was a real and stalwart barrier to help-seeking. As important as it is to understand the sources of youth's psychological pain, it is equally important to understand why youth and their families struggled to access appropriate help for that pain. If nothing is done about the hurdles to help-seeking that we uncovered, any intervention to address youth's psychological pain will remain incomplete and ineffective. Children will continue to die by suicide. Not all of these problems are unique to Poplar Grove—similar barriers to mental health help-seeking are noticeable in communities across the United States—but as a collection of barriers, they fundamentally disrupt the effectiveness of any efforts at suicide prevention in ways that leave local youth vulnerable to suicide.

4.1 WE KEEP IT QUIET

Throughout the United States, and in many societies around the world, mental health problems carry stigma, which makes it hard to talk about them publicly.[3-6] By this, we mean that mental illness is perceived as a character flaw indicative of a person's failings,[1,7,8] rather than a medical problem or a painful struggle deserving of respect and support. Instead of being cared for during their suffering, the individual is blamed as incompetent for not being able to control their own behavior or emotions or take care of themselves. We glimpse this stigma when people tell depressed individuals to "snap out of it" or just be happy. These perhaps well-meaning but ignorant phrases imply that our psychoemotional state is completely under our control, rather than recognize that mental health problems are often more profound than that, rooted in our genes, our biology, our history of trauma and social pain, as well as the rules, expectations, and social norms present in the places we call home.[9] Yet even if the person hearing "just snap out of it" understands the true complexity of mental illness and psychological pain, these comments can sting. The power of stigma is its multipronged attack. Whether we want to or not, it can be quite challenging not to internalize, at least to some extent, cultural beliefs about our personal experiences with mental illness or mental health struggles. And when we internalize these beliefs, even if only partially or unconsciously, that in turn can lead to imagined or anticipated blame from others, in addition to real judgments we may experience.[8] We quickly learn what others think about someone with a mental illness and begin the process of hiding that part of ourselves to avoid being judged, because we can anticipate just how people will react to the knowledge under the specter of mental health stigma.[10,11] We don't expect kindness or the encouragement of help-seeking; rather, we expect judgment and blame. Importantly, social blame and judgment—or even just the expectation of it—often leads to deep shame.[12,13] And not for nothing, shame is one of the emotions that is associated with higher risk for suicide.[14-16]

Sociologist Erving Goffman was among the first to identify and investigate the toxic patterns around stigma.[7] He argued that possessing a stigmatized characteristic essentially spoils a person's identity. It becomes that person's dominant trait, the one thing that defines them in others' eyes and sometimes in their own. And that strips them of the dignity of being seen as they want to be seen—as complex people, full of multiple traits and identities, like daughter, student, athlete, animal-lover—reducing them instead to being mentally ill.[1] In this scenario, regardless of how amazing a person is, regardless of how many wonderful ways they contribute to their communities, possessing just one stigmatized trait can ruin it all.[7]

To be clear, mental health stigma is a cultural belief that many people, including those still spreading stigmatized beliefs, can easily reject as erroneous. Mental health problems are prevalent in the United States, and many of us will deal with these problems at some point in our lives. They are also increasingly prevalent among youth,[17] signaling the importance of pushing back against negative cultural perceptions. To actively support all aspects of youth well-being, we need to teach kids about mental health fitness and destigmatize mental illness.[4] Yet we noticed Poplar Grovians frequently used language indicative of stigma when we asked about youth suicide. They spoke of mentally ill children as being a "blemish on the perfect . . . family," "deviant," or "mentally deficient." They said mental illness was a "taboo" topic that revealed a "fatal flaw." And they said "it"—that threatening "it"—wouldn't happen to my family, to a good family.

Jim's insistence that his son Ian was "normally a good kid," truly, just not when he was having one of his "episodes," was unsurprising in this light. He needed to preemptively defend Ian's goodness because, as we heard numerous times, even the medical professionals and mental health workers in Poplar Grove regularly referred to kids with mental health problems as "not good" kids or not "normal." "This was not a healthy girl," one mental health professional shared of a local teen who died by suicide. "This was *not* a wonderful girl. This was a girl with serious mental illness." While the person who made these comments may not have meant to communicate stigmatizing messages—they may have just meant that she was just not the happy-go-lucky kid people saw her as—this is ultimately beside the point; that is, whether the person meant it or not, these comments are loaded with judgment, blame, and shame. The implication is that one cannot be both a wonderful person *and* someone with a serious mental illness. And when this is articulated by the very professional meant to help with mental health struggles, this message can be incredibly hurtful. No wonder it was hard to be honest about "having issues."

If mental health was talked about in Poplar Grove, it was usually after a tragedy cracked open the silence and created space for disclosures and conversations—sometimes life-saving. In those moments, we can see both the potential for change, for a different way of seeing mental health and help-seeking, *and* the stigmatizing beliefs that, as we will show later in this chapter, likely contributed to the tragedy. After Aria died, her family's sudden willingness to talk about mental illness really changed the dynamic of their friend group. "We're really close with the [Stephens] family," said Hugh, a family friend and dad to one of Aria's childhood friends, Parker. He continued:

> The one thing that has come out [after Aria's death] is that [her family is] candid. It's open. The Stephens have really taken it a step farther, and [are] making sure that people are just talking about mental health issues, and that it's ok to talk about them . . . So that instead of it being, "Oh my gosh, this is something you keep behind closed doors, this is our problem, and it's kind of embarrassing to share," instead, it was, like, "Hey, we are a village—let's be here for them and let 'em know we all have eyes on this situation." . . . [and Aria's] dad [Will] came forward and said that he'd been bipolar his whole life. We didn't know that, but he's not a man of secrets, but it's not really something you would just candidly share with anybody.

Hugh's surprise at the Stephens's new candor reveals that silence was the norm, though friends and neighbors seem to have been very kind after Aria's suicide. For the first time, they learned that their friend Will had a bipolar diagnosis. It's rare to be candid about "something" so stigmatized. All at once, spurred by Aria's death and encouraged by Will and his wife Josie's disclosures, families in their intimate circle of friends began to talk about how they were struggling with the same things. "We actually had a friend in our group who [was] having problems with their daughter," Hugh recounted. The conversations started by Aria's parents, "made them realize that they should probably get counseling for her. And it was okay to talk about it." Breaking the silence was literally an exceptionally positive aftereffect of another terrible loss. It shows us how the tide can be turned on mental health stigma.

4.2 CONTACT WITH MENTAL HEALTH PROFESSIONALS

While Jim felt unsupported by the mental health professionals he interacted with, and while we heard stigmatizing talk from mental health professionals, this was only part of the story. The mental health professionals—including therapists, clinical psychologists, social workers, school and crisis counselors, family medicine physicians, pediatricians, emergency medicine physicians, and psychiatrists—that we spoke with in Poplar Grove reported that their most salient on-the-job challenge working with kids was the pressure from parents to keep it all quiet. In other words, they felt the effects of mental health stigma, too. "I have worked with families whose children have been seriously mentally ill and needed to be hospitalized for a number of different reasons," began Walter, a mental health professional. "Children who have been cutting themselves and depression and a whole host of other things probably. And the feed-back I've gotten from those parents . . . [is], 'we're covering it up, we're covering it up.' 'It's going to be fine.'" Fellow mental healthcare worker Jocelyn attributed the coverups to "the stigma of getting help." As she put it, "It's the, 'My kid doesn't need help, you know, he's just being a kid,'" pattern. Jocelyn continued:

> Well, families don't want to recognize it for themselves, they don't want to recognize it for their kids, kids don't want to tell about their parents having issues. . . . And I think part of the dilemma for us [as mental health workers] . . . is that there is a stigma associated with getting help, mental health in general.

This stigma made it really hard to get "parents . . . to recognize [the] signals and signs" of psychological pain among their children, remarked Carina, a mental health worker: "I think parents around here don't like to think their kids are not alright, and so, they're like, 'oh, let's keep moving along.'" This pressure to pretend appeared when kids were nearing a serious crisis. Bill, a mental health professional, agreed:

> As professionals, we try to get the parents on board with [addressing their kids' problems] but they don't want to deal with it. I think that's my biggest issue. You can see the red flags all over the place and the parents don't want to do anything, even to the point to where kids can even threaten to kill themselves and you call [the parents] and [they say] "oh they're just playing around," or [I'll call and say] "I think you need to take them in . . ." [and they'll respond] "oh they'll be perfectly fine."

Just as it was shocking to read in the previous chapter that Aria knew help was an "easy" reach away and accessible through multiple people, it is shocking to hear mental health workers in Poplar Grove talk about how hard it is to get parents to take mental health seriously and get their children to a hospital when necessary. This is a town with an excessive suicide problem. Yet parents like Josie and Will, who had been worried enough about Aria to talk with her about depression in the week before her death, had never insisted Aria seek mental health help. In retrospect, Josie acknowledged, "That's one of the things I really wrestle with."

Obviously, this situation isn't great for kids, but we were hearing that it was also extremely stressful for mental health workers. "It just tears you up inside," Bill added. It also meant that along with treating kids, Poplar Grove's mental health workers have to put a lot of effort into educating parents. A clinician named Christine articulated her approach to the prevalent mental health stigma as centering the support and teaching of parents as a major part of children's therapy. She shared:

> I think parents need a lot of support. In my work, I work heavily with parents. And not necessarily the same way that I'm working with the kids in terms of helping them with their struggles. But [parents] are my co-therapists. They are the ones I need to empower, and build

coping, and support for them, whatever. And I am just always so touched by the depth of commitment and caring to their kids. And as educated as they might be, as psychologically minded as they might be, as willing as they might be, sometimes blinders are just up. And without any intentionality whatsoever, and to have that outside person to kind of be able to do that more with them, I think at the end of the day makes the whole process stronger.

Like Christine, we found that parents in Poplar Grove loved their kids fiercely. They were highly committed to doing everything they knew to do to raise happy and healthy adults. When we talk about suicide in Poplar Grove, we are *not* talking about unloving or bad parents any more than we are talking about bad kids. The problem is that parents—like all people—often rely on their long-standing cultural beliefs about good parenting, mental health, child development, and so on, while they try to navigate new conditions or challenges, like a child's anxiety, depression, drug or alcohol abuse, or suicidality. These cultural beliefs are so deeply ingrained that parents cannot always recognize when their ideas about how things "ought" to be are holding back their ability to support their child through what simply is. Cultural beliefs thus lead some parents to perceive a child's self-harm not as a sign of serious distress, but as "an attention-seeking thing," as one informed a child that we interviewed. Or to say to their suicidal and depressed child that "it's not really a big deal . . . just get over it." Or to deny the child's experience and say, "Oh, you're not depressed; you're just having a rough day." The "it" is so unthinkable and unspeakable that parents distance themselves and their families from "it" rather than turning toward the problem.

Our society more generally,[1,18] and Poplar Grove specifically, does not welcome conversations about mental health, and so parents do not easily encounter opportunities to change their beliefs without the intensive support and guidance of therapists like Christine. Parents like Jim, however, felt that in their moment of need, they *didn't* find themselves in front of patient, dedicated therapists who could take the time to educate them. Other parents may not be ready or able to hear the guidance offered by mental health professionals. Everything, no matter how gently said, may sound like blame when it has to do with the deeply stigmatized problem of mental illness.

4.3 WHEN MENTAL HEALTH ISN'T TAKEN SERIOUSLY

Predictably, the silence around mental health has serious consequences. Mental health workers were concerned they were seeing kids too late— after the kids were already in crisis. They also felt like parents wanted fast solutions so they could end their contact with mental health professionals as quickly as possible. This meant that parents didn't always stick with therapy or recommended long-term treatment, potentially undermining a kid's ability to heal and ultimately be well. Robert, a mental health worker, found this really stressful:

> When we do see kids, there's this crisis, and [the parents are] kind of like . . . "Fix my kid" and the participation from the parents [isn't optimal] and that's when it happens that the kid doesn't see any kind of change [in their family]. We see that a lot, we have a lot of that happening where they want us to fix the kid, there's a crisis situation, and then after two or three sessions they go away, and you call them up and say "don't you want to continue to do this until you resolve this all?" and then they wonder why their kid is struggling again.

If we imagine this scenario from the perspective of the teenager in need of and trying to access help, the full consequences come into focus. Many youth describe extraordinarily frustrating experiences with mental health help-seeking. No matter how many suicide losses happened in the community, young people felt that parents didn't always take their mental health struggles seriously Recall the parent who spoke of suicidal ideation as a cry for attention rather than a serious signal of emotional pain. Similarly, when Madison shared in a teen focus group that *"parents don't care!,"* including her own parents about her own self-harm, her contemporaries, Hannah and Lily eagerly agreed that this is a major issue. The students quickly began speaking over each other.

HANNAH: They don't take it seriously . . .

LILY: Personally, right now, I'm dealing with this one friend of mine. She's more like an acquaintance. She's self-harming, and I've been pushing her to get help. And the first thing I did before even pushing her to get help was to tell her mom what was going on. You always think that when you tell their parents, they'll be like "Oh my gosh, please don't hurt yourself." I pushed this girl to get help from her mom, and, maybe it's this town, maybe it's that she's Latina. My grandpa is Hispanic, and there's, like, stigma against mental health. [The girl's mom] started yelling at her, screaming. They had a worse relationship because of it. [Her mom] sees it as an attention-seeking thing. It absolutely doesn't matter if she's hurting herself for attention or hurting herself because she wants to hurt herself.

HANNAH: Either way, there's an issue. If you would hurt yourself for attention, regardless, there has to be something bad enough that you need attention. There's something *wrong*. Even if you're faking being sad . . . that wouldn't happen . . . because why would you . . .

MADISON: My friend . . . he was feeling really suicidal and depressed and no one would talk to him about it. He would try to tell his parents, his grandmother's brother, but he just kind of ignored him, and put it off like "Oh, you're just sad because you're sad." And then once he started self-harming, they were all like "Oh my gosh! What's wrong?" If you're just sad on your own, it's not really like a big deal because it could just be that you're sad. You're not like . . . *ill*. You don't have an illness. You're just sad that day. Like, get over it. It's like telling someone who has depression "Just get over it." Like you have a cold. Go take medicine for it. And you'll get better. Sleep it off. You'll get better. And it doesn't really work like that.

HANNAH: It's like telling someone with a heart condition to "make your heart work right" or something.

MADISON: Yeah. It's like telling a person with cancer, "Stop." [Everyone laughs] That's basically what it is, 'cause I've had people tell me "Stop being so sad." And I'm like, "Wow, *thanks, Doctor Obvious!* That's great advice!" It's not like I try to do stuff that take my mind off of this stuff *all the time*. It just, doesn't work. It's not like I *try or anything*. Do I just sit in my room, in the dark, all the time, and listen to sad music, and play the violin? No. I do things. I do normal everyday things, I'm with people all the time, and they don't know. And I am happy *sometimes,* and I am not happy other times, and I can't control it half of the time. So, it's just kind of one of those things.[i]

Amid the perennial adolescent pastime of trash-talking parents, these are big problems supported by the systematic agreement of Poplar Grove's mental health workers. We would, perhaps, push back again on the idea kids raise that "parents don't care," but the teens were correct that parents can misunderstand how serious something is or how hard it is to change one's emotions. Josie and Will Stephens cared about and were aware of their daughter's distress, but their daughter's depression, oversleeping, and not showering didn't necessarily make them think "This could be suicide!" So they did not take urgent action. When we don't take early signs seriously, we miss opportunities to connect a youth who is sleepless, or sleeping too much, or avoiding social activities they used to enjoy to potentially life-saving resources.

For a full list of warning signs or risk factors for suicide, visit https://afsp. org/risk-factors-protective-factors-and-warning-signs. Additionally, to get training in identifying warning signs for suicide and to learn how to talk to people who may be at risk of suicide, we recommend LivingWorks trainings (we have no affiliation with this organization, but use their trainings ourselves): https://www.livingworks.net.

Another concern here is that scientific research demonstrates that youth who have a trusted adult in their worlds—be it a family member, mentor, coach, or school counselor—experience better mental health outcomes, more willingness to seek help when things get difficult, and less vulnerability to suicidal thoughts or attempts.[19,20] But youth have to be able to talk about mental health with those trusted adults for this potentially life saving help to be effective. Among the youth and young adults we interviewed, this was borne out: having the support of a therapist, parent, or adult mentor that they could talk to about anything, including mental health, was, simply put, a game changer. As we saw in Chapter 3, when parents or adult mentors provide authentic help, it can be an extremely powerful and positive experience for youth. It was often adults who paved the way for cultural rebels to find their peace and build lives that felt worth living despite tremendous loss and grief, social and academic pressures, and mental health challenges. Scott, one of the cultural rebels, responded to a question about coping with feelings around not living up to Poplar Grove's expectations for youth by noting simply, "[I] talked about it with my mom." When asked, "That helps a lot, huh?", Scott—always succinct in his responses—was again matter of fact: "Yes." College student Molly pointed out that "for teenagers, probably one of the only ways to start getting help is to like talk to your parents about what problems you're having." Shara concurred: "Just where do you go in Poplar Grove to get help on mental health unless you tell your parents? Nowhere."

In truth, adults are lucky when they find out about their child's mental health struggles. It can be all too easy to overlook small signs of distress, just as Josie and Will Stephens didn't realize the small signals of distress that Aria was revealing were, in fact, indicative of substantial psychological pain and risk for suicide. It can be hard to recognize these signals for what they are. This disconnect is an important aspect of how mental health stigma generates silence, suppresses crucial help-seeking, and contributes to the suicide problem in Poplar Grove. Kids learn a lot from adults, parents, and beyond, absorbing their cultural norms. That includes whether and when to talk about mental health and what it means to have mental health problems. Often, Poplar Grove's kids concluded they were supposed to keep it under wraps. "In Poplar Grove, everything is supposed to be perfect: good grades, good kids who go to good colleges. All the bad stuff gets covered up," said teenaged Hannah. "Nobody wants to be like, 'I have an issue.' And nobody wants to come out and be honest about [their issues]. So kids cover it up and try to act like they are doing well in school and they are being the Poplar Grove kid that they are supposed to be." Isabel, a young adult concurred: "We have to be this perfect little town, and we have to be good at everything, and everyone has to be good at everything, and you can't talk about things that are wrong."

Being the Poplar Grove kids that they were "supposed to be" was top of mind for the youth we met—a fact that some adults seemed to grasp. And it was just as salient to the ways kids thought about and approached help-seeking in Poplar Grove. "Some people are gonna judge," Natalie confided, so when sometimes "it gets too dark . . . when you're that deep in a hole . . . you don't want to reach out to other people." The pressure to be what other people want, what other people expect, mattered, and youth understood that it was always possible that private information about mental health could easily slip out into the public domain. No one wanted to take on the label of mental illness. "I know a lot of my friends who've like gone to therapy before," Madison shared, "and one who has gotten on a new medication recently. The school finds out the next day, and [then] everybody knows. You can't really trust anyone [not] to tell. . . . And then, everyone knows, and they're like 'What's wrong? What's wrong? Why do you have meds?'" These could be expressions of care, yet it was the fear of judgment, fear of everyone knowing, and fear of not meeting expectations that figured so heavily in the suppression of help-seeking in Poplar Grove.

4.4 A SPOILED IDENTITY

As Erving Goffman, that foundational sociologist, would predict, these fears all traced to stigma. They changed how youth saw their own lives and evaluated their self-worth, with fundamentally important consequences for their help-seeking. "The hardest thing for me to accept today," Felicity confided when reflecting on her near-fatal suicide attempt as a teenager, "is that I didn't give my friends a chance to be there for me." Now secure and happy as a young adult, Felicity described her teen years surrounded by a wonderful group of friends who dubbed themselves "the Super Friends."

Many are still close friends. "It was . . . the network that you would want a young girl to have. I was [also] in a youth group at Grace Community Church and we would do retreats . . . it was . . . so special," Felicity shared.

And yet, when Felicity's mental health began to deteriorate, she never reached out to those friends, she never confided in them how terrible she was feeling. "Was I able [to reach out to my close friends]? *Yes.* Did I? *No,*" Felicity declared. "The thought [of telling my friends] never crossed my mind. . . . It wasn't like I had a debate and said, 'Oh, I've got to tell Lizzie how I'm feeling, but I'm embarrassed.' Or, 'She's going to think less of me.'" Instead, help-seeking just "wasn't who [I] was." Felicity explained:

I'm not the type of person [to ask for help] . . . I did kind of go to my friends and talk to them about my frustrations [and fights] with my mom in particular. So I feel like they were there for me then, but when it came to all the other stuff, again the loss of enjoyment, being sad for no reason, feeling judged and all the other stuff, I never thought "I'm feeling—like something's really wrong and I have to talk to someone. Why don't I tell my friends?" . . . I know they would have been there for me, there's no doubt.

Like Aria, Felicity was aware that her friends would have been there for her, as they were when she needed to vent about her mom, but unconsciously, the story may be more complex. From a young age, Felicity said, she learned from her family and the community that having a mental illness was at odds with being, in her words, "a good person" and with being a kid that lived up to community standards. Indeed, though Felicity later came to understand her mother as living with diagnosed bipolar disorder, when she was younger she regarded her mom as a "bad person" who was "crazy" (her direct words). Her mother earned these labels through explosive, angry, public outbursts and serial infidelity, which Felicity learned about at a young age. As Felicity told us:

I judged my mom. I think as a young child when you hear something [about your mother] there's [just] good and bad. It's like "my mom's a bad person. My mom cheated on my father." Maybe [as an adult you think] maybe there's a reason. Maybe things are hard. [But as a child] you don't think like that. It's like "okay, my mom is now a bad person" . . . I lost respect for her . . . I had this judgment against my mom that she's a bad person and now she's acting crazy, so that's because she's *not a good person.*

When Felicity's friends and her father repeated these judgments about Felicity's mother, it reinforced Felicity's impression. While it may be typical for a teen's friends to call her mom "crazy" for her outbursts and unpredictable nature, her father could have chosen his words and selected his confidant more carefully. One time, when Felicity was a child, she sat with her father in their church parking lot as he cried over the state of his marriage. She asked, "Why don't you divorce her? . . . She's doing these things. Why do you keep letting her do this to you?" As she remembered, he replied, "I just love her so much. I just love her . . . [and] that makes things more complex." Felicity's father tried to explain to her that her mother was a "sick individual" and, though Felicity felt like it was unlikely they had a clear diagnosis at the time, she understood what her father meant: "mentally, she was not right." He would tell Felicity, "She's sick. She's demented in the way she does things." The message the girl received was "She doesn't think straight." It was a painful situation for a child experiencing one adult's instability and manic episodes, another adult's ongoing pain, and the deep sense of community control.

As a young adult, Felicity came to understand her mother's behavior as a symptom of mental illness. She regretted her youthful judgment and has come to respect her parents' marriage. Back then, though, she was a kid in a community defined by strict norms about ideal families and a penchant for gossip as a mode of teaching and imposing those norms. Felicity recalled feeling intense embarrassment as a teen that she "didn't have a sane mom," more so even than having a mother who engaged in infidelity. "Now . . . I know she has an illness," Felicity said in hindsight. "But as a child, it was like 'oh my gosh, I have this crazy mom!' And it was sort of embarrassing because again, the things she would say . . . [and] the drama she would cause."

Stigmatizing beliefs about mental illness loom large in this narrative, particularly as Felicity turned to talking through her own suicide attempt. She continued using language that emphasized being "good" or "bad" as a person. For instance, when explaining why she never sought help, Felicity shared:

> The best way I can explain it is it's kind of the person I became. I don't know if this goes back into that mentality of where I was just like, "I gotta be a good person," where I just sort of became the person I was known as and then I saw myself as this strong, independent person [who] didn't need overprotective parents. I didn't need anybody guiding me. I was like, "I'm a leader. I know what I'm doing. I'm good at solving problems. I'm good at listening." There were all these things that again I kind of prided myself on.
>
> Looking back now, like I said, I did sort of get this righteous feeling going back again comparing to my mom. It's just like, "I'm such a cool person," and again, this self-esteem of "I've got this." . . . Again *I* was the advice giver. *I* was the one—*I* wanted to be that role model again that people came to versus—I wanted to always have the answer. I think I always had this feeling—going back to that righteous feeling—like if I didn't have the answers, nobody else did.

Much of Felicity's decision-making process around help-seeking, then, had to do with her understanding of herself and what people like her did and did not do. Fiercely proud of her independence, competence, and "goodness," she was "not the type of person" to admit she didn't have the answers and needed outside help.

Interestingly, the psychological pain and depression—as she came to understand and label her experiences during her psychiatric hospitalization after her suicide attempt—behind Felicity's suicidality *also* felt at odds with who she was. They felt like a coordinated attack on who she was as a person and her ability to meet her own and others' expectations. Felicity was absolutely an ideal-typical Poplar Grove student—star actor, top achiever, go-getter, role model. Felicity and her peers, who we spoke with, saw her as such. "I was very set in who I was and very proud of who I was," Felicity asserted. But "losing her mind," losing her ability to achieve, let alone function, made her fear she was losing it all. She confided:

> [Before my suicide attempt,] I can remember a specific thought. I can't actually remember if I drew it or if I just visualized it in my mind of a—it was almost like a bar graph. I remember thinking of a container where I feel like I've always been at the top of the bar graph or the container of intelligence. I was always kind of a step ahead of everyone in intelligence and what I'm doing and getting things and being a leader.
>
> And then it was like, I remember feeling like I feel like, "I'm down here now [gesturing down]. Everybody else is up here [gestures up]. They're sitting in math class getting these hard problems and making sense of it. They're getting it. They're intelligent." And I'm feeling like—I remember feeling stupid, like, 'I can't comprehend this stuff,' where again, all through my life, I was the go-getter. I was the smart one. I got things. It was always about making sense of things. I made sense of things. . . .
>
> I felt like I was losing not only my mind, but myself. I talked a little bit about how I prided myself on this righteousness and being good, but I think *I also prided myself on intelligence because again, comparing to my mom, I thought she was crazy.* "She's insane, she doesn't think rational thoughts."

Felicity's psychological pain brought intense exhaustion and brain fog. It challenged her ability to concentrate, to learn, and to think rationally. As she began to struggle in math class, the somatic complaints she'd later recognize as depression symptoms felt dangerously like her mother's irrationality was bubbling up inside her. It was, in her mind, bringing her dangerously close to *being like her mom*, being "crazy," being a "bad" person. Felicity's depression spiraled. As she recounted:

So, it was like, I got a lot of anger towards myself when I'd be like, "What's wrong with me? Why am I not here [gesturing up on her invisible bar chart]?" . . . My grades were slipping, but it was like I just wasn't functioning as a human being . . . and that's when the low self-esteem kicked in because then I started—I'm feeling like "okay, I'm not getting stuff in math class. I can't stay awake. I'm feeling overly sensitive with one of my friends . . ." I would start to compare myself more to people then too, because it was, again it was low self-esteem.

In Felicity's experiences, we see how generalized beliefs about being an ideal person can be interpreted as incompatible with mental illness, or even just psychological pain. Felicity owned these beliefs, turning them on herself as she believed her beloved community would do. Viewed through this lens, alongside all we already know about Poplar Grove, it is easy to understand why Felicity interpreted her symptoms not as experiences that could pass with time and supportive therapies, but as indictments of her goodness. What she saw as a fundamental flaw in her personhood felt so enormous that it rendered her entire self worthless.

Felicity's experience illustrates how an identity can become spoiled. Recall, realizing that a person possesses a stigmatized trait can essentially cause them and others to see the person as ruined. In this context of strict cultural beliefs, mental health stigma, and where all eyes *are* on you and word travels so fast, the sense that a flaw is both plain and insurmountable is immeasurably painful. Spoiled identities often trigger intensive perception and behavioral management.[2,21] Meaning that in contexts ripe with mental health stigma, people often try to hide the fact that they are suffering and spend precious energy managing other people's impressions of them rather than getting help for their pain. This process of impression management and hiding psychological pain can be exhausting and mentally taxing. It requires hypervigilance and a finely tuned sense for any sign—real or imagined—that others have caught on to their "secrets." Since Felicity had firsthand experience of her mother's struggles and the moral judgments placed upon her, it is not surprising that it literally never occurred to Felicity to ask her parents, or her friends, or her pastor for help. She could maintain her public persona as a "good person" while complaining to friends about a stressful or even embarrassing family situation, but felt her own worth would be challenged (or, in the moment, that what she saw as her own worthlessness would be forever exposed) if she spoke about her own mental health troubles. Admitting to needing help was more painful than finding another way out of the situation. Suicide seemed better, from Felicity's perspective at that time, than crying out for help.

Not surprisingly, when Felicity returned to Poplar Grove High School (PGHS) after her psychiatric hospitalization, she felt herself sliding right back into her suicidal despair and exhaustion. Being back in high school around all her peers was just too much. She ended up transferring to a small, private school in a nearby town to finish up high school away from the pressures of PGHS. In this alternative context, she thrived. She went on to a great college and, eventually, a great career. But ideally, returning to her school and her friends wouldn't have been "too much."

4.5 THE SHAME TRAP

Felicity was caught in something we call *the shame trap*. Shame is a painful social emotion that feels as if you do not, in some egregious way, belong to your community—broadly defined.[22] This is why shame is considered a social emotion. Absent a reference group, absent other people who might judge us, shame, like guilt and pride, would not exist. Social emotions emerge when we evaluate ourselves and our behavior in comparison to the social expectations of people who matter to us.[23] Shame's social purpose is as a quiet, intense emotional warning that we are at risk of being cast out of a valued community, that our secret is a threat to our social survival. Being resoundingly rejected—ostracized—by a social group we care about (even if we do not necessarily *like* the group) feels dangerous and enormously painful. The intensity of this pain and fear is something sociologists call a social death. We need our people, our community, to survive, and when we feel those people might be slipping away, that they might hate or despise who we are as a person, it can feel like our very survival is threatened. Fear of something like social death is enough to generate internalized pressure to conform to community expectations[24]; the pressure is identical in intensity to the risks associated with not fitting in, meaning it's extreme in Poplar Grove. In moments when conformity feels impossible, we feel our shame rising. We feel trapped, like there is no way to regain self-worth and social acceptance.

The conditions are right in Poplar Grove for things like social death and the shame trap to be real and powerful in people's lives. The cultural beliefs in the community are widespread, broadly shared, well-known, and largely taken for granted as "natural," "right," or "obvious." It's hard for Poplar Grovians to imagine different answers to the question of why wouldn't parents want their children to be top achievers? Why wouldn't parents want the "best for their children"? Poplar Grovians therefore have a high incentive to regulate their own conformity to those shared and internalized beliefs, no matter how hard they find that effort. After all, thanks to the dense social networks, the risk that one's deviations from cultural expectations will become widely known via the grapevine is extremely real.

It's also key that we realize shame is relative. It can come no matter how small the infraction might seem in other communities with less stringent prohibitions against particular identities, behaviors, or experiences. Still, being able to see how other communities handle particular characteristics in less stigmatizing ways can be a powerful protective factor for people not in those communities. Being exposed to diversity of opinions can help people akin to our cultural rebels in Chapter 2 to navigate, resist, or make up their own minds regarding how they feel about who they are, and how they feel about mental illness and mental health struggles. Unfortunately, in Poplar Grove, the vast majority of youth explicitly commented they had little sense of what it was like to be a kid anywhere else. They struggled to know what was a universal truth of growing up in the United States and what was something more specific to growing up in Poplar Grove.

Understanding this general aspect of mental health stigma and the shame of a (perceived) spoiled identity is helpful as we work to understand why youth die by suicide. Shame hides in plain sight. It's difficult to talk about, sometimes hard to name or recognize, but it's so often a factor in the lives of families in Poplar Grove.[25]

To be sure, we never saw a case of families, or Poplar Grove as a community, casting out a child for any reason. But we saw a lot of evidence that kids *felt* they could be rejected. Many youth were desperate to stop the suicides and ensure the safety of their friends, yet they thought it was inconceivable to admit to their own mental health struggles. Shame and spoiled identities can help us understand Aria's fundamental and emphatic objection to seeking help, though she was offered help and understood more help was easily available. Having a mental illness was, for her, inconceivable as a part of a life worth living—no matter that she lived with a father who was living a happy, full, and "successful" life while taking medications to manage his bipolar disorder. The profound stigma of mental illness and the shame trap it created had made suicide a less painful option than help-seeking in Poplar Grove. Between a threat of social death for feeling like they didn't fit in and literal death by suicide as a way to escape their pain, too many kids were opting for the latter.

4.6 CONCLUSION

According to the Centers for Disease Control and Prevention, depression, anxiety, and other mental health problems are fairly common and rising among US youth. Many mental health advocates, healthcare providers, and scientists like us argue that mental health problems must be taken as seriously as, and be perceived no differently than, physical health problems. They warrant healthcare, concern, and support. There is absolutely nothing shameful about having mental health problems or seeking help for psychological struggles. We don't mind revealing that we, your authors, are no strangers to psychological struggles and are grateful to our therapists who provide critical psychological support. We aren't alone. Globally, about 10% of people will experience depression.[26] This impacts so many of us, and yet so many of us are embarrassed about going to therapy or having a mental health diagnosis.

We saw this in Poplar Grove where youth—and their parents—found it hard to seek help for mental health problems, which contributed to the disproportionate rate of suicide in this otherwise idyllic community. Unfortunately, a corollary to the culture of great expectations and "perfect" kids and families in Poplar Grove was a denial of any mental health struggles or psychological pain motivated by prevalent mental health stigma. Kids and families felt they could not meet community expectations *and* have a mental illness or experience psychological struggles. This pattern is rooted in mental health stigma or the idea that having a mental health problem is a character flaw of the gravest kind—an imperfection— rather than a normal if painful part of human experience. Instead of help-seeking, "embarrassment" was a common reaction to experiencing a mental health problem. To avoid the judgment of others or to avoid feeling painful emotions like embarrassment and its close cousin shame, kids and parents in Poplar Grove avoided talking about mental health issues, including with mental health professionals. It was better to keep it quiet, to keep it private, than to seek out potentially life-saving care. This reveals how we can't preach help-seeking without also making sure we're ending mental health stigma.

Social movements are trying to address this by encouraging the normalization of mental health help-seeking. Aria's family is currently at work in Poplar Grove with new allies doing this work, changing the conversation by role-modeling that mental illness isn't shameful. Yet stigma is very sticky. And when it suppresses help-seeking and treatment, we can end up with tragic outcomes and tepid responses. Unfortunately, the same forces that stymied help-seeking during suicide prevention mattered to how the community, particularly the school, responded after youth died by suicide, revealing yet another layer of the onion that we must peel back to understand the suicide problem in Poplar Grove.

NOTE

i. We connected Madison to mental health care after this exchange, care that she stuck with for years.

REFERENCES

1. Link BG, Phelan JC. Conceptualizing Stigma. *Annual Review of Sociology.* 2001;27:363–385.
2. Link BG, Phelan JC. Labeling and Stigma. In: Aneshenel CS, Phelan JC, Bierman A, eds. *The Handbook of the Sociology of Mental Health.* New York: Springer; 2013:525–541.
3. Martin JK, Pescosolido BA, Olafsdottir S, McLeod JD. The Construction of Fear: Americans' Preferences for Social Distance from Children and Adolescents with Mental Health Problems. *Journal of Health and Social Behavior.* 2007;48(1):50–67.
4. Pescosolido BA, Perry BL, Krendl AC. Empowering the Next Generation to End Stigma by Starting the Conversation: Bring Change to Mind and the College Toolbox Project. *Journal of the American Academy of Child & Adolescent Psychiatry.* 2020;59(4):519–530. doi: 10.1016/j.jaac.2019.1006.1016.
5. Phelan JC, Link BG, Stueve A, Pescosolido BA. Public Conceptions of Mental Illness in 1950 to 1996: What is Mental Illness and Is It to Be Feared? *Journal of Health and Social Behavior.* 2000;41(2):188–207.
6. Thoits PA. Resisting the Stigma of Mental Illness. *Social Psychology Quarterly.* 2011;74(1):6–28.
7. Goffman E. *Stigma: Notes on the Management of Spoiled Identity.* Englewood Cliffs, NJ: Prentice-Hall, Inc.; 1963.
8. Corrigan P, Watson AC. The Paradox of Self-Stigma and Mental Illness. *Clinical Psychology Science and Practice.* 2002;9:35–53.
9. Abrutyn S. Toward a Sociological Theory of Social Pain. *Journal for the Theory of Social Behaviour.* 2023;53(3):351–371. doi: 10.1111/jtsb.12371.
10. Binnix T, Rambo C, Abrutyn S, Mueller AS. The Dialectics of Stigma, Silence, and Misunderstandings in Suicidality Survival Narratives. *Deviant Behavior.* 2018;39(8):1095–1106.
11. Perry BL. The Labeling Paradox: Stigma, the Sick Role and Social Networks in Mental Illness. *Journal of Health and Social Behavior.* 2011;52(4):460–477.
12. Scheff T. Shame and the Social Bond: A Sociological Theory. *Sociological Theory.* 2000;18:84–99.
13. Abrutyn S. Toward a General Theory of Anomie: The Social Psychology of Disintegration. *European Journal of Sociology.* 2019;60(1):109–136.
14. Lester D. The Role of Shame in Suicide. *Suicide and Life-Threatening Behavior.* 1997;27(4):352–361.

15. Abrutyn S, Mueller AS. The Socioemotional Foundations of Suicide: A Micro-sociological View of Durkheim's Suicide. *Sociological Theory*. 2014;32(4):327–351.
16. Wiklander M, Samuelsson M, Asberg M. Shame Reactions After Suicide Attempt. *Scandinavian Journal of Caring Sciences*. 2003;17:293–300.
17. Lake AM, Kandasamy S, Kleinman M, Gould MS. Adolescents' Attitudes About the Role of Mental Illness in Suicide, and Their Association with Suicide Risk. *Suicide and Life-Threatening Behavior*. 2013;43(6):692–703.
18. Schnittker J. Public Beliefs about Mental Illness. In: Aneshenel CS, Phelan JC, Bierman A, eds. *Handbook of the Sociology of Mental Illness*. New York: Springer; 2013:75–93.
19. Singer JB, Erbacher TA, Rosen P. School-Based Suicide Prevention: A Framework for Evidence-Based Practice. *School Mental Health*. 2019;11(1):54–71.
20. Wyman PA, Pickering TA, Pisani AR, et al. Peer-Adult Network Structure and Suicide Attempts in 38 High Schools: Implications for Network-Informed Suicide Prevention. *Journal of Child Psychology and Psychiatry*. 2019;60(10):1065–1075. doi: 1010.1111/jcpp.13102.
21. Chaudoir SR, Earnshaw VA, Andel S. "Discredited" Versus "Discreditable": Understanding How Shared and Unique Stigma Mechanisms Affect Psychological and Physical Health Disparities. *Basic and Applied Social Psychology*. 2013;35(1):75–87.
22. Scheff T. *Emotions, the Social Bond, and Human Reality*. Cambridge, UK: Cambridge University Press; 1997.
23. Tangney JP, Steuwig J, Mashek DJ. What's Moral About the Self-Conscious Emotions. In: Tracey JL, Robins RW, Tangney JP, eds. *The Self-Conscious Emotions*. New York: Guilford Press; 2007:21–37.
24. Shott S. Emotion and Social Life: A Symbolic Interactionist Analysis. *American Journal of Sociology*. 1979;84(6):1317–1334.
25. Cohen D. The American National Conversation about (Everything but) Shame. *Social Research*. 2003;70(4):1073–1108.
26. Lim GY, Tam WW, Lu Y, Ho CS, Zhang MW, Ho RC. Prevalence of Depression in the Community from 30 Countries Between 1994 and 2014. *Scientific Reports*. 2018;8(1):2861. doi: 10.1038/s41598-41018-21243-x.

5

THE SCHOOL'S
POSTVENTION RESPONSE

*I probably remember that day, like, more vividly than any other
day in my high school career. Like, better than graduation, better
than prom.*

—Gwen

Molly was stunned. As a normal Tuesday became one of the worst days
of her life, she could only sob in the corner of her gym class. She'd just
learned her best friend Michelle had died by suicide the night before.[i] She
remembered later that the gym teacher told the students they could go to
the school counselors' office if they needed support, but "I just sat there,
and all I was doing was crying . . . I was in shock. I sat there for an hour
and a half during gym, just crying." When gym ended, Molly trudged to
the locker room. She didn't want to go to her next class. "But for some
reason, it didn't occur to me that I didn't have to go. [That] I could go to
the guidance office and leave school like all of my other friends had done
that morning." Instead, Molly dutifully went to her next class—advisory
or "homeroom"—where it was business as usual. "We were supposed to
vote" on the prom king and queen, Molly remembered, "and I was just
staring at the paper. . . . I was just not there. I had tears in my eyes . . . [but]
everyone around me is chatting because it's not a real class." This teacher,

who had known Molly all throughout high school, noticed the girl's tears as she collected the ballots. She stopped and, in an authoritative voice, told Molly, "You should go to the guidance office." It was precisely what Molly needed in that moment. "She didn't even ask if I wanted to [go]. She was just like, 'You should go . . . do you need someone to come with you?'" Hours after the devastating news, an adult finally took charge, *took care* of Molly, and let her know how to access some measure of support and comfort. In the years since, Molly reflected, "I've always been really grateful to [my teacher] for doing that."

It's impossible to underestimate youth's emotional vulnerability after a suicide loss. Youth grieve, but without the life experience and emotional resources of adults. Kids also have reactions every bit as varied and complex as adults, from self-blame to anger to an urge to memorialize and mourn collectively. Youth often experience suicide losses at least partially within the context of school, where the sometimes judgmental gaze of peers is ever present and teachers are often focused on the business of learning rather than on kids' social-emotional well-being. Imagine that, like Molly, you've just learned your best friend is gone, and your teacher is still leading gym class, as if you're not in the corner sobbing, or that your peers are chattering, teasing, and voting for prom king and queen. Or imagine that you weren't very close to Michelle, but you are an empathetic teen, or a teammate, or sat behind her in math, or have experienced another recent tragedy that triggers strong emotions at the news. Suicide losses in schools hit everyone differently. And that's appropriate. Grief is a complicated business. But for some, a suicide loss can upend everything, making how the school operates that day critical to taking care of kids.

Crisis responses focused on suicide losses are often referred to as suicide "postvention," and when the losses are among youth, schools are a key site of response. Suicide postvention specifically encompasses the activities and organized interventions undertaken to limit suffering as much as possible, promote healing, and prevent additional suicides.[1] Schools' postvention strategies can greatly shape how the loss of a young person impacts the student body. Indeed, schools are the most critical place where youth can be connected to help[2,3] and where the vulnerability that accompanies a suicide loss[4] can be addressed. Indeed, if there is any hope of encouraging the help-seeking we know is crucial yet frequently downplayed in Poplar Grove, schools must establish a comprehensive evidence-informed plan for suicide postvention before a suicide happens.

So how did Poplar Grove High School (PGHS) respond to suicide losses? With this chapter, we take up this question, the answer to which is critical to understanding both the suicide problem in Poplar Grove and how to enact compassionate, caring postvention that supports youth on what can be one of the most devastating days of their lives. But before we begin discussing postvention at PGHS, it's worth taking a moment to discuss how difficult postvention can be for US schools.

5.1 THE CHALLENGE OF POSTVENTION

At this moment in the United States, we collectively ask a great deal of teachers, counselors, and other school staff. In addition to providing students knowledge through age-graded curricula, we expect school staff to protect kids in myriad ways—as mandated reporters, they are asked to spot the signs of abuse and intervene; as classroom heads, they must take charge in nightmare scenarios such as natural disasters or active shooter incidents; and as informal confidants and advisors, teachers are supposed to balance school policies, children's well-being and intellectual lives, and parents' often unstated but strong preferences. And all this as budgets and resources are slashed. The expectation now is that schools also should be competent at suicide prevention and, if needed, postvention.[5] Yet this is a new and still developing role for educators—as it is for everyone else. The first comprehensive suicide postvention guide for schools, *After a Suicide: A Toolkit for Schools*,[6] is just 13 years old at the time of this writing, and scholars point out that there remain substantial gaps in the scientific understanding of how to prevent and respond to school-age suicide losses.[2,7-9] Poplar Grove was well into its struggle with youth suicide before best practices had been communicated for responding to the problem.

Even when schools have a well-thought-out suicide postvention plan based on evidence-based guidelines,[3,5] actually leading a school through the aftermath of a suicide loss is no easy thing. Balancing many different people's needs, preferences, and capacities means there are almost always those who are unhappy with what the school does and does not do. There isn't a "right way" to do suicide postvention; this is part of the challenge. Even the most detailed guidelines today often only provide general considerations rather than clear instructions. One guidebook cautions schools that "it is particularly important to avoid idealizing the person and glorifying suicide," but gives no examples to clarify the difference between memorializing or remembering and idealizing or glorifying a student or their death.[2 (p. 8)] When it comes to memorializing students, the book continues, schools are asked to "focus on how the student lived, rather than how he or she died,"[2 (p. 26)] though taking that approach may romanticize the death or sow confusion about suicide and its causes. In short, guidebooks appropriately reflect the complexity of the situation, and they leave a lot of room for interpretation and discretion when it comes to best practices about postvention. How, for instance, should a school day proceed as the news of a suicide loss spreads throughout its classrooms and community? Schools are left to interpret these guidelines on their own, ideally with guidance of local mental health experts.

The difficulties of school-based postvention go beyond scarce resources, competing responsibilities, and unclear guidelines. Schools must also take into account privacy laws pertaining to minors, differences in the ways staffers interpret guidelines, families' wishes, and the unpredictable responses of their students. For instance, what if a group of kids organizes an impromptu vigil at the school, which is discouraged by evidence-based guidelines? Should the school ignore the gathering, send a crisis response team to participate (potentially making it seem like the school endorses the event), or risk ordering kids to disperse and head home? This latter option is likely the poorest choice, as it does not communicate authentic caring, which can be really painful for teenagers in the face of a loss, yet it may comport with the school's policies. It also sends kids off to grieve alone, far from professional help. (For what it's worth, we would probably send the crisis team). Schools are in a bind, too, when it comes to sharing information publicly about a student's death. Privacy laws are one thing, but so are the wishes of the bereaved family—who may yearn to avoid the stigma associated with the cause of death or who may just prefer privacy—and the needs of the community, which may not understand why the school cannot talk more frankly.

Simply put, suicide postvention is very difficult for schools. We ask so much of them on tragic days, and we rarely acknowledge how much is beyond their control, and how vague existing guidelines are. When guidebooks are followed in real life by real people with their own cultural beliefs and biases and with their own talents, needs, emotions, and limitations, the end result rarely matches the original guidance.[10] How faithfully a school's postvention conforms to recommendations depends, in part, on the specific staff who undertake the response. When school staff are not trained to talk about suicide, or when they are not trained in how to help students in the aftermath of suicide, they can easily make mistakes. It takes training and preparation to avoid mistakes about this uncomfortable topic, to avoid upsetting students or causing inadvertent harm,[3] and to look for students in need of further help. We see some of this in Molly's story, in which her gym teacher fell short but her advisory teacher came through in a moment of real need.

Another simple truth: the science is still limited on which school postvention strategies best promote healing.[8] Our society generally does not support grieving people well or talk openly about death or loss, let alone suicide and mental health.[11] And even under the best of circumstances, schools can't control everything. We can almost guarantee that some part of a postvention effort will go awry. As we discuss school responses to youth suicide in Poplar Grove and how they sometimes caused kids pain, we need to hold tight to our purpose. All this is to learn and improve, not to blame and shame grieving kids, schools, or communities.

5.2 ACKNOWLEDGING THE PAIN

Poplar Grove High School did a lot of things right during their postvention responses. They frequently brought in crisis counselors from the school district to support students, and later, they began to bring in a county crisis team to support school staff's mental health needs. They had School Resource Officers (SROs)[ii] coordinate incident command, organizing the practical realities of crisis response—space, food, and connecting to community resources. Still, PGHS's postvention over the years of its suicide clusters was fraught with challenges and barriers to the provision of authentic care.

The greatest issue kids cited with the school's response was their generalized sense that the school just didn't care. "Our school administration just kind of pretends it's not there," teenaged Leah shared. Her sidekick Kaitlyn quickly chimed in, "Yeah, that was really kinda wrong." Leah continued, "They just didn't talk about [Quinn's suicide], like, at all. They had, like, one moment of silence the day of and that's it." Shannon, who was also deeply impacted by Quinn's death, felt the school wanted to erase Quinn's existence: "In first period, the day after it happened, my teacher didn't even mention it. . . . The teacher didn't even say one thing about it [despite the fact] that there was literally an open seat [Quinn's seat] right next to me." Shannon's mother agreed, telling us, "It was like [Quinn's suicide] didn't happen," like the school said, "'We're moving on.'"

Guidelines suggest returning to "normal" school routines as quickly as possible, but that felt dismissive and hurtful for many youth. Quinn's death substantially impacted the school community, and it was not the first suicide Leah, Kaitlyn, and Shannon had been through. Though the girls had repeatedly seen PGHS experience a suicide loss and then, to their minds, return to business as usual, it remained shocking to them.

The feeling that PGHS moved on too quickly was present across the years and across the suicide deaths. It was a constant postvention complaint in our interviews. Recalling when her classmates died by suicide, Isabel, one of our older young adult respondents, speculated that the school community didn't want to "face that we weren't perfect" and "so many things [got] swept under the rug. . . . [The school] just doesn't want to be seen as anything less than perfect." Vanessa, who experienced Michelle's suicide, used similar words:

People here, they, like, think it's sad and everything, but then they just kind of like dusted [it] under the rug, like it didn't even happen. And then, when it happens again, they just do the same thing, and they just, like, don't really acknowledge it. And they don't do what they need to do about it because nobody is educated enough about it. So I don't know, I just feel like they need to have a better grip on what's going on and not be like, "Oh," just, "Another one happened."

Collectively, these sentiments suggest that schools can move on too quickly, and that when they do it can convey the message that kids' deaths, and thus their lives, don't matter.

5.2.1 The Need to Talk

One of the challenges with moving on and getting back to "normal" is that it runs contrary to kids' need to process and talk about what has happened, their need to understand and figure out what to do next. Isabel lamented that she and her classmates were never "encouraged to talk about [the suicide loss]. Even our teachers didn't talk about it. It was like, 'Alright, let's learn geometry.'" In truth, Isabel didn't really *want* to talk about suicide, which to her was "very scary and very big." But Isabel needed to talk:

I more so wanted to talk about what it was like to be in high school at the time, because I felt like a lot of adults didn't understand or maybe didn't want to understand, or maybe just didn't believe us when we said, "We're stressed out!" . . . "This is really hard!" and "We're really scared!" They were like, "Oh, you're fine. It's just high school." But it's so much more—and people are dying! This is a big deal—this anxiety, this depression, this whatever it is is very real.

With striking eloquence, she finished, "I wanted to talk about *that*, [about] what it was like to *live* in Poplar Grove rather than to die here."

By not talking about suicide much after a suicide loss, we end up denying the reality of kids' existences, their concerns for their peers and for their own lives and futures. We also shut down conversations about help-seeking, about mental health, and indeed, about signs of suicide and suicide prevention. For many students, this was the crux of the problem.

This need to talk and process and remember that many impacted teenagers have after a suicide loss is both quite normal and at times problematic. One of the most important charges of postvention is to not romanticize or glorify suicide. Schools' practical approach to this directive is frequently not to allow memorials, vigils, or even group conversations centered around the student who has died. And while we agree that memorials or vigils at school can be unsafe, because they can so easily slip into glorifying suicide, denying students these rituals made some of them quite angry, even years after their losses. In the face of Shannon's anger, we asked what she thought PGHS could have done better. "I guess I would want a little bit more recognition," Shannon replied. "There was a really big feeling of feeling like we weren't remembering her enough." Shannon was adamant she hadn't needed more information on suicide risk factors, but a sense that Quinn's mark on this world was permanent. "Let's just put up a freakin' plaque with her name, in the school, and leave it there," Shannon exclaimed. "It's not a huge thing to ask for, but it's saying, like, you know, now she's not just buried six feet underground somewhere. She was here, and she was part of this, and she existed here." To Shannon, these were just obvious steps in *remembering* Quinn, her too-short life, and why she mattered.

The school, however, had adopted the official stance of the American Foundation for Suicide Prevention and their collaborating organizations:

While there is no research to suggest that permanent memorials create a risk of contagion, they can be upsetting reminders to bereaved students. Whenever possible, it is recommended they be established off school grounds. The school should bear in mind that once it plants a tree, puts up a plaque, installs a park bench, or establishes a named scholarship for one deceased student, it should be prepared to do so for others, which can become quite difficult to sustain over time.[3] [(p. 30)]

The school district thus advised Poplar Grove schools to not "let students display any type of shrine" or "plant a tree, t-shirt, or plaque, etc." We generally agree with these guidelines and understand the school's stance. But instead of redirecting Shannon to some other shared space in the community where a plaque might be placed, the high school just shut down Shannon and her friends. As Shannon told us, "They were like, 'That's too in-your-face.'" She continued:

> It's like [the school] is so worried about the waterfall effect with the next person happening, that they don't even do anything to remember the person who was gone. And that was just really frustrating, and that was a major source of my anger and a lot of other people's anger— was, like, "It was something that had happened!! Talk about it! Do something about it!" I mean, I'm not saying, "Who cares about," like, "it triggering another person," but it doesn't matter if it triggers the next person right now, 'cause that's not what we're focused on. We're focused on these hundreds of people that are now sitting here crying to bed every night, 'cause she's just gone, and they didn't even get to see her one last time, 'cause the casket was closed.

Like many young Poplar Grovians that we spoke with, Shannon desired the school to acknowledge the pain and suffering she was experiencing around her friend's death. Remember, the school is one of this community's strongest institutions, a focal point for kids and adults alike. Its choices are consequential, well beyond its walls. Shannon's words also caution us to remember grieving kids and their needs—these very kids are most vulnerable to developing suicidal thoughts or attempting suicide after the loss of a friend or a peer.[4,12]

Shannon was correct that the school was extremely concerned about what she called a "waterfall" effect, which is more often referred to as a "ripple" or "contagion" effect. Our interactions with school representatives were marked by palpable concern that their actions might trigger more suicides. We witnessed community members vocally blaming the school for past suicide clusters, so the school seemed to do anything and everything to avoid any chance that a student's death might be glorified or romanticized and thus trigger a new suicide cluster. Remembering felt *dangerous*. A PowerPoint summarizing crisis response in Poplar Grove's school district acknowledged this could make the postvention "feel less caring" and more "awkward," but cautioned, "You do not want to spread suicide contagion." This makes us sad. It is not right for a suicide postvention to feel more awkward or less caring than any other crisis response or response to a student death. Students' pain and suffering cannot be met with chilly awkwardness.

We explained our concerns about memorialization at school to Shannon in our interview, in part to see how she responded. Shannon got it. Interrupting our question, she declared that suicide was, in fact, "glorified." She continued:

> That's what I was even telling people, too . . . I know what you're saying. It's like, [what if a kid is feeling like] "I want to die because I feel like nobody loves me," and all of a sudden looking up [at a student's memorial] and being, like, "Maybe that is my [answer]." It's illogical, but, "Maybe [suicide] is my step to being loved and being remembered."

Shannon's reaction when we nudged her to see the broader picture—the array of concerns the school is supposed to balance—illustrates something we saw repeatedly in our research. Kids can be serious partners in suicide prevention, eager to keep their peers safe and remember those they've lost. But hey need information. They need to be taken seriously. They need to have their voices heard. When those things happen, safe and respectful postvention is possible.

Shannon's response also reveals the importance of acknowledging suicides whenever possible and as soon as possible when they occur. When the school cannot confirm that a particular kid died by suicide, it is still necessary to talk about suicide, particularly if it is widely known that someone died by suicide despite the family's desire to keep that information private, as is quite common in our experience. It really harms students when important adults seem dismissive about suicide. As bereaved families have a fundamental right to control the narrative about their child's death, it's wise for schools to speak regularly with students about mental health and suicide, decoupling the topics from any one child's death or periods of intense mourning. Of course, in Shannon's case, Quinn's family was immediately forthcoming about her cause of death, meaning that the school made active choices to not talk openly about her suicide when they could have. We wonder whether youth would even feel a need for a permanent memorial if frank, emotional conversations about suicide could happen in the wake of a fellow student's death. The thing kids appeared to want most was for their peers who died by suicide to be remembered—for a kid like Quinn to *matter*.

5.2.2 On Empty Chairs

There is one way that teenagers do not want their friend's absence memorialized: through an empty chair in a classroom seating arrangement. Several youth, like Shannon, specifically mentioned the pain of staring at an empty seat. Whether it was meant as a respectful gesture or staff were just not attuned to the need to shift seat arrangements upon a student's death, PGHS students and grads alike found the practice upsetting. "I had three classes with Zoe the semester she died," Rachel remembered with a grimace. She continued:

> None of the teachers even thought to rearrange the freaking seating in the class! Like, I stared at her empty chair for a month. And, that was really . . . Like, thinking back on it now . . . Those silly little things, like, everyone missed. And, like, how impactful that was to be in that setting where no one really knew how to deal with it, and something as simple as like, "Hey! Let's switch up the seating for the

class of the rest of the time" so I'm not literally staring at an empty chair for a month. You know?

After a Suicide recommends that seating assignments should be rearranged about a week after a student's death. They also suggest that teachers discuss this with students and explain "in advance that the intention is to strike a balance between compassionately honoring the student who has died, while at the same time returning the focus back to the classroom curriculum."[3] (p. 28) This way, students may also have some say in the rearrangement: "For example, they could read a statement that emphasizes their love for their friend and their commitment to work to eradicate suicide in [their] memory."[3] (p. 28) School staff might use the visual absence of empty chairs as a reminder that, in this intense period after a loss, they must stay attentive to the many small reminders throughout the school day that can cause moments of pain for everyone in the school community. In our own personal experiences as professors communicating with the students in our classes about the loss of a classmate, we try to prioritize honoring the deceased student, communicating compassionately, and then carefully redirecting the class back to the material at hand. Being honest, compassionate, and communicative, taking the time to explain why you are doing what you are doing, goes a long way toward helping students feel like their experiences matter, no matter how indirect or direct the impacts of the loss might be for each individual. Making students feel like they matter is critically important during postvention.

5.3 THE ROLE OF TEACHERS

Teachers are the front line of schools' suicide postvention responses. Their tasks are challenging, and some proportion of the teachers in a school will need to seek crisis counseling themselves. In fact, a process for bringing in substitute teachers should be a part of any school's crisis plan. Among these tasks, the first may be to deliver the news of the death to their students.³ Ideally, teachers will be given a statement to guide them through talking with the class, as well as evidence-based information to share when talking about suicide, facts about suicide, warning signs for suicide, and guidelines on what to do to seek help in a crisis.³ In directly impacted classrooms, and in those where a teacher does not feel comfortable breaking such news to their students, a trained crisis counselor (a mental health professional) or other staff member can take on or assist in the task, answer questions in an appropriate and nonstigmatizing way, and provide support to those who need help in the moment. When we do not train school staff to talk about suicide, loss, grief, or mental health, which was the case during our fieldwork in Poplar Grove, these tasks become immeasurably harder.

Teachers are a school's "eyes and ears." Because they have the greatest chance to see which students are struggling and connect them to care, they are essential to the mental health safety net. Unfortunately, PGHS teachers did not seem to have clear guidance on how to support youth, which led to gaping holes in those safety nets. Most likely, most teachers fell somewhere in the middle between the teacher who seemingly ignored Molly's distress at the start of this chapter and the one who recognized it and authoritatively connected her to much-needed supports. In our interviews, students often spoke fondly of their teachers, how they saw the pressure kids were under and told them that they mattered. But without training, even teachers who cared inadvertently communicated harmful or stigmatizing messages about suicide. For example, Madison said that after a series of repeating suicides, "a lot of the teachers take it to heart, and then I know from my advisory teacher, he talks [about mental health] all the time. We have the same things about bullying and self-esteem every year for advisory. And, he always talks like, 'Yeah. You're selfish if you kill yourself.'" She scoffed at her advisory teacher's comments, adding, "That's probably the worst thing in the world to say to somebody!" But we heard about similar teacher interactions throughout our fieldwork, and students often agreed with Madison that the idea their classmates were "selfish" denied those kids' very real suffering and blamed them for having problems that, as Madison felt, were caused by other people.

Regardless of her teacher's intent, Madison was correct that his approach is not considered part of helpful suicide prevention messaging. Dr. Stacey Freedenthal, a leading expert in the clinical treatment of suicide, explains in an excellent essay titled "10 Things Not to Say to a Suicidal Person"[iii] that the "suicide is selfish" statement simply "inspires more guilt" in a suicidal person. If our greatest concern after a suicide is promoting healing and help-seeking to ensure that no additional suicides happen, we should take great care to realize that any child we are speaking with could have suicidal thoughts. And speaking to them in a stigmatizing way could exacerbate their vulnerability to suicide. We'd add that statements like these further suggest that the adult in question has not built the capacity to empathize with the experience of teens, and teens desperately need empathy in the wake of a suicide loss. A better alternative for any moment, but particularly during postvention, is for adults to ask how kids are doing, then listen to their answers. When kids mention things that cause them pain, teachers—or anyone, really—should make an effort to validate their feelings rather than tell kids they are selfish for considering suicide. Anyone can learn to effectively talk to kids about mental health and suicide, but it often does take some guidance and training. Such training would help us all overcome stigmatizing attitudes about mental health or suicide and make sure we don't perpetuate myths about suicide. Talking about suicide becomes one more thing that we must ask teachers if they can do, because we need them to.

5.4 THE STRUCTURE OF CRISIS COUNSELING

If teachers are the eyes and ears, crisis counselors are the heart of postvention. They play the most critical caring role, as distressed youth are sent to them for help on what is likely one of the worst days of their young lives. While we were not able to speak to many youth who found themselves face to face with the crisis counselors, returning to Molly's story can help us identify points for improvement in crisis counselors' work in schools.

When Molly's advisory teacher sent her to speak with the crisis counselors, Molly faithfully took herself down to the school counseling office. Typical of her other interview comments, Molly noted that Michelle's suicide was a "really difficult situation" for the school as well as for her, while admitting the counselors hadn't provided much help at all. Molly shared, "When I went down to the guidance office that day that everyone found out, I talked to this woman. I was just all over the place. I was crying. I felt like she didn't really get what I was saying and just didn't really realize that I was actually really good friends with Michelle." That issue alone is worth unpacking.

Identifying students who may be highly impacted by a suicide loss is included among *After a Suicide's* guidelines for schools.[3] But it is a tricky business. Schools generally begin by trying to identify family, friends, teammates, clubmates, and classmates, and that's what PGHS did. Teens on the list were to be pulled from class and brought to the school counseling office. One difficulty with this method is that adults in school buildings are not always aware of the intricacies of students' social relationships— another reason why teachers, as the school's eyes and ears, are so crucial. PGHS encouraged all students to self-report to the counseling office, but some, especially if they noticed other students being called to the counseling office for support, got the message that somehow they didn't "deserve" support, that their grief didn't make the cut, no matter how upset they were. That was part of Molly's experience:

MOLLY: I felt like I didn't have the authority to give myself the permission to [go to the counselors] because when I was in gym, someone from the guidance office came and took a girl who played lacrosse to the guidance office specifically. I guess that really confused me, because I was like, "Why aren't they calling me down specifically? I was on her team." I didn't play lacrosse but—

ANNA: Yeah, you played soccer with her.

MOLLY: I did! So why aren't they calling [the soccer team] down specifically? But they didn't, and that really just confused me. I was already—I don't know. I was just like, "I shouldn't go down there.

I'm not one of the people who deserves to go down there." I don't even know.

It seems that Michelle's beloved lacrosse teammates made the list, but her soccer teammates, for whatever reason, did not. This was particularly painful for Molly, who was also extremely close friends with Michelle, though they were in different grades at PGHS. All schools have to make these lists in a hurry, and almost certainly, they will miss some students. The point is that not having her name on the list actively discouraged Molly from seeking help and made her need for support feel illegitimate. That sense was compounded when Molly finally found herself in front of a counselor who seemed, to Molly, confused by her grief—presumably because Molly was not on the list.

Again, no school is going to perfectly create a list of impacted students in the aftermath of a suicide, and crisis counselors can sometimes get overwhelmed by the number of students who need help and the kinds of help they may need. Molly's scenario does, however, invite us to consider the structure of crisis counseling. Lists are necessary, but imperfect, and it should be made clear to all involved that students who are not on the list may still be highly impacted. Additionally, kids in distress do not need adults to question the closeness of their relationship to the person who died or the intensity of their emotions. Grief is complicated. Being nonjudgmental and responding to kids' emotions in the moment, with evidence-based interventions and supports, is very important.

We highlight the importance of having well-trained crisis counselors as well as school counselors, social workers, and psychologists, who often support schools during crisis and who know what to say and how to support kids, because Molly's experience wasn't isolated. Riley, who was close to several youth who died as part of a suicide cluster, had her own painful experience with the counselors when her friend Braden died. "I remember going to the [counseling] office," Riley recalled. "I think I was called [to the office] because the counselors were trying to figure out if Braden's death was on purpose or not. There were some people talking, and they were like, 'Do you think it was a suicide? Do you think he took all those pills on purpose?' Then I was all angry again." Riley was extremely impacted by Braden's death, and from her perspective, this intervention made her life worse, not better (no matter the counselors' intentions in that moment). It is not appropriate to use youth to try to understand why their friend died or to determine whether it was by suicide. That is a job for the medical examiner or coroner, not the school and certainly not a student weathering gutting news.

The effectiveness of crisis counseling may also be supported by being thoughtful ahead of time about the physical setup. On the day of Michelle's death, PGHS was overwhelmed by students' needs. All students seeking help were sent to the student counseling center where Vanessa, a student in Molly's grade, said she arrived "still in shock, still not crying, and, like, everyone around me was crying. And like the whole, like, counseling center was just filled with people." Given Poplar Grove's cultural penchant for gossip and the stigmatization of help-seeking and mental health challenges, the public nature of seeing a crisis counselor—the fact that it meant entering a crowded space with grief on full display—could be its own barrier for help-seeking, especially for tentative kids like Molly or others who knew they didn't make the list.

The crowd in the counseling office also created other challenges. Vanessa, in part, went to see the counselors as a way to support her best friend, who was extremely close to Michelle. Unfortunately, that aspect of her experience was not positive either:

So, I was, like, sitting there, like, looking around for my friend. She was, like, in a back room, basically a storage room, and there probably were, like, 10 kids [in there]. And, like, the teachers were yelling at us for, like, for leaving the [main room]! And everybody was just sitting in there crying [with staff], like, telling us where we can and cannot go. And they were like—they got, like, very sassy about it. They were like, "Well, what do you want us to do?" And we were like, "Can a big group of us just go outside and sit on the track?" Like, we're not going anywhere, just let us, like, go somewhere where we can breathe. I don't know, I just feel like they had no idea how to handle it, and they just kind of like—I don't know. I felt like they treated us like aliens. They were like, "We don't know what to do with you guys."

It's easy to imagine that, in the face of overwhelming need, the school's capacity to keep track of kids and to provide the ideal one-to-one ratio of students to crisis-trained counselors was severely strained. And yet the school's job is not only to connect kids to crisis counselors, but also to keep track of them, to keep students safe. From the school's perspective, it was risky to let kids wander around, processing their emotions anywhere. Indeed, from a suicide postvention standpoint, that would not have been a best practice. At the same time, kids need an emotionally safe place to process their emotions, and that may not be in a crowded counseling center, surrounded by peers, where their grief feels like it is placed on public display.

The frustration that Vanessa felt likely resulted from this clash of responsibilities—the competing needs of the school and its students. Ideally, schools could quickly swell staff numbers so that, in this moment, when kids most needed empathic adults and schools most needed to keep track of distressed kids, youth could get the individualized care they need without feeling like they were being "treated like aliens." Many districts temporarily swell staff members during a crisis by borrowing crisis-trained school mental health staff from other schools. Safe spaces and calm, competent adults who are trained to help kids regulate their emotions and figure out what they need to be as okay as possible in the moment are essential to an ideal response. Making sure that enough staff flood the school so that kids can be supported through diverse mechanisms is crucial, too. Some kids may need to go home with family. Others should not go home, even if they want to, if at home they will be alone. Still others may need a private place to cry, a crisis response-trained mental health worker to debrief with, or the ability to stay with peers for group-oriented interventions. Space is at a premium in many schools, so we recognize that this may be a tall order, but it seems wise to plan ahead and anticipate the need for multiple spaces and responses. When youth are impacted by a suicide loss, it may be time to prioritize crisis response over business as usual and co-opt otherwise needed spaces for crisis counseling. Using technology already widely used in schools and during crisis responses (e.g., walkie-talkies and electronic forms), it should be entirely possible to diversify the structure of crisis counseling while also keeping track of kids and keeping them safe.

The conclusion of Molly's story of the day she learned of her loss provides our last caution for crisis counseling: never overlook follow-up. "When I was leaving [the counseling office]," Molly remembered, the counselor "was like, 'We're going to call and check up on you in a week or two,' or something. 'You can come back in.'" And yet no one called. As Molly described:

> They never contacted me at all in any way, shape, or form. I always thought that that was very—I don't know why they never did . . . I felt like that should've been their responsibility to call me in and ask specifically how I was doing. . . . Maybe that lady didn't write down [to follow up with me] and then no one saw [my name on follow-up lists], or she wrote it down, but no one did [anything]. I don't know how it failed, but no one in the counseling center ever did any follow-up with me.

It was hard for Molly to seek help and the lack of follow up damaged her trust in her school. "I don't know if I felt neglected, but I felt like they forgot about me, they don't care. They're not making the effort to make sure I'm okay. I really didn't like that, because I wasn't okay." Molly didn't connect with counselors again until college, years later. Today, she's an amazing, caring, thoughtful young adult, yet the intensity of her grief and the other challenges she faced in her personal life suggest that she would have really benefitted from additional contact with counselors and psychological supports during high school. If the crisis counselor or the school's counseling center had followed up with Molly after Michelle's death, they would have realized her distress that day was not a brief, temporary emotion, but grief that would follow her for years. They may have connected her to out-side psychological care and saved her years of struggle. The plethora of painful emotions that typically follow a suicide loss—like grief, anger, fear, and guilt—do not disappear overnight, and so it is expected that some number of students will need further grief counseling in the community. Because they spend so many hours at school, however, schools should also continue to play their role in mental health safety nets by following up with affected students after their loss and providing families with guid-ance in connecting to any needed community resources.

5.5 INEQUALITIES IN RESPONSE

There was one more theme that stood out in our interviews on the schools' postvention responses to suicide. Youth noticed significant inequalities in how the school responded to different student deaths. *After a Suicide* fully endorses tailoring postvention to the details and circumstances of an indi-vidual suicide loss,[3] as does PGHS's district. We, too, accept the necessity of tailoring responses. One way that responses get tailored is according to the number of students impacted by the death. The more students are counted as impacted, the bigger the response is likely to be. For example, after Michelle's death, the counseling office was overflowing. There was no way to avoid that or to support students without sending more crisis counselors, which further amplified the apparent intensity of the response to Michelle's death. But in a place so concerned with social status, it is worth hearing how the differences in the way peers' deaths were treated in the school sometimes made kids feel.

Recall that Riley, a student, lost several friends (Lauren, Braden, and Forrest) and a classmate (Kennedy) to suicide and drug overdoses that occurred as a cluster. She felt crushed when she compared the school's ap-parent reaction to Kennedy's death and its reaction to Braden's a year later. "They didn't say anything about Braden on the announcements,"[iv] Riley began, "but they did for Kennedy." She continued:

Kennedy's death was a huge deal in Poplar Grove. I remember going to class [the day of Kennedy's death] and, like, teachers were crying, and they were like, "Go to the auditorium. There's counselors there if you need to leave class and talk to somebody because you can't deal with being here." There was nothing like that for Braden. He wasn't a popular kid. He was definitely not a "Poplar Grove kid"—like the stereotypical [guy] or whatever. He was a little bit chunky. He didn't have a whole lot of friends, but we all cared about him so much. Like, he was a great kid . . . [I was so] offended [by the difference in response]. Because—I know Kennedy was involved in the school and all the extracurricular activities and whatnot, but Braden was still a student there. Just because he wasn't a smart kid or super involved in the school system doesn't mean they shouldn't say anything. He was still here. So many people just didn't realize or have any idea. I just walked down the hallway, and it's just another day to everybody else [while] I'm like, "My whole fucking world is falling apart. I don't understand."

The main thing is that this young person took the perceived magnitude of the school's response as evidence of how much Braden and Lauren mattered to the school compared to how much Kennedy mattered. We cannot and should not try to control the emotions expressed by teachers and students. They are simply one element of a response a school can't control, but they do figure into the degree to which a death feels like huge news versus just another day. Perhaps if the school had focused on supporting Riley, rather than pumping her for information about Braden and what she knew about his mental health, this young person wouldn't have felt Braden and Lauren's deaths were less important to her school than Kennedy's. Again, making students feel supported and acknowledging that their grief and their friend's death, whatever the cause, could go a long way toward heading off this additional pain.

It's also possible that Riley's reaction reflected broader inequalities in community responses to the youth suicides and overdoses. We noticed that the popularity of the deceased student affected Poplar Grove's overall response, both in our interview data and in our own observations when youth died by suicide during our fieldwork. Likewise, kids whose deaths could be easily explained by widespread stereotypes about suicide seemed to make few waves.[13] Aaron, for instance, was widely thought to be abusing drugs and alcohol, and thus his suicide somehow "made sense" and was only a minor blip on the community's radar—quickly communicated to the town's resident sociologists, but seemingly forgotten a week later— while Aria's "shocking" suicide was discussed extensively and for weeks, if not years. PGHS is tightly coupled with the community, and its responses to suicides are vitally important beyond its walls. One key takeaway is that, to the extent possible, suicide deaths should be treated similarly, re-gardless of estimates of "impacted students." Care must be taken to not in-advertently imply that one child's death matters more or less than another, whether due to their social standing or the cause of their death. Indeed, we always recommend—as does the American Foundation for Suicide Prevention—that whatever a school does to memorialize the passing of one student or staff member must be the same for all students or staff members, regardless of the cause of death. To do otherwise is to convey that some deaths matter more than others and that is antithetical to au-thentic caring.

5.6 CONCLUSION: HOPE FOR THE FUTURE

Suicide postvention is one of the most challenging tasks that a school can take on. Even when following all of the best guidelines that science can offer, the reality is that schools are asked to balance individual students' desires and needs with the needs of the whole school community. Understandably, this can leave some students feeling hurt. In the time after our fieldwork in Poplar Grove, we've had the opportunity to watch several schools respond to suicide losses. Many had copies of *After a Suicide: A Toolkit for Schools* and adhered to its principles, yet postventions still sometimes left people frustrated, even angry. Over our years researching in Poplar Grove, we were heartened to note substantial improvement in a number of aspects of the school's postvention responses, despite the fact that many of our young interlocutors and their parents felt that PGHS remained woefully inadequate in that regard. For example, PGHS stopped notifying students of losses over the public address system and started being more thoughtful about its messaging to students and families.

The most consistent limitation to PGHS's crisis response during the time of our study was its ongoing hesitation to talk about suicide directly for fear of causing a suicide cluster to form. It seems that many of the choices the school and its district made were motivated by this sense of risk. The guidance from Poplar Grove's school district as recently as 2017 was to "not announce [or confirm] the death was a suicide," regardless of the family's wishes. The district also warned school staff that "you do not want to spread suicide contagion" by doing things differently than the guidelines suggested, but confoundingly added a caution that schools and teachers should not "sweep the nature of the death under the rug." The school seemed to us to be genuinely concerned that talking about suicide, or confirming that a given death was a suicide, might *cause* suicide. Perhaps administrators simply thought that if a suicide loss wasn't confirmed, there would be no possibility of inciting a suicide cluster. These are both myths. As stated at the outset of this book, talking about suicide does not cause suicide.[14] And students have so many ways of discovering the truth about a peer's death that any effort to deny that a suicide has happened is essentially moot. In short: the school's evasion of suicide as a topic likely made its community *more* vulnerable to suicide clusters, rather than less.

The avoidance and silences, our interviews revealed, frustrated youth, alienated them from school staff, and increased their feeling that the school just didn't care. Collectively, these things weaken school-based mental health safety nets and further depress help-seeking, something already stigmatized by the community's cultural norms. After their bad experiences, students like Molly and Riley were unlikely to seek out their school's counselors ever again.

We urge school administrators, staff, crisis counselors, and others who find themselves leading a postvention to remember that their first and foremost role is to be authentically caring for youth. Communicating, explaining, listening, collaborating, and providing sufficient resources are all key to building authentic, meaningful relationships between youth and adults that create safety and care, no matter the magnitude of the tragedy.

Since our time in Poplar Grove, we see reason for hope. After 2017, legislation mandating the regular training of teachers and other school staff in suicide prevention has swept the United States.[5] By 2021, similar laws[v] that require "all educators in the state to complete at least 2 hours of youth suicide awareness and prevention training each year in order to be licensed to teach"[5] had passed in 21 states. This legislation, which the American Foundation for Suicide Prevention supports, aims to increase a school's capacity to "identify students at risk" and to "ensure that students at risk are assessed and evaluated by a mental health professional (within or outside the school setting), according to school protocol or policy."[5] We argue it actually does so much more: it provides an official avenue for state and local governments to say youth suicide matters and to acknowledge that schools are expected to do this work and need support, resources, and training to do the job well. Currently, this legislation is often unfunded, which means that once again we are increasing schools' responsibilities and obligations without providing resources, yet the spirit is important. The state in which Poplar Grove resides passed some of the most comprehensive legislation, mandating annual training in suicide prevention for teachers and other school staff. That development came after our field-work ended, and so we do not have information about its effects at the school level—still, we can't help but feel a little hope.

NOTES

i.   Unfortunately, Anna didn't ask Molly how she learned the news. We only know that
     she learned it at school. We often choose to not interrupt our interviewees when
     they are sharing very emotionally fraught parts of their stories. This unfortunately
     means we sometimes miss details that we realize later would have been helpful to
     know. From other students, we know that it was not over the announcements.

ii. SROs are police with special training to work in schools—while their main job is
     to prevent school violence, they often do play a role in mental health safety. They
     are sometimes the only professionals in school buildings who can veto a parent or
     legal guardian and require a child gets crisis mental healthcare. Police (though not
     usually SROs) are also often the individuals who perform after-hour welfare checks
     on children who may be suicidal.

iii. Dr. Stacey Freedenthal's essay "10 Things Not to Say to a Suicidal Person" can be
     read here: https://www.speakingofsuicide.com/2015/03/03/what-not-to-say/.

iv. It is not recommended to announce student losses over the intercom system. Many
     kids reported that they learned of suicides over the announcements; however, the
     school stopped doing this before our fieldwork started, perhaps because of the
     chaos youth reported in earlier incidents.

v.   Sometimes called, as a group, the Jason Flatt Act.

REFERENCES

1. Andriessen K, Krysinska K, Kõlves K, Reavley N. Suicide Postvention Service
   Models and Guidelines 2014–2019: A Systematic Review. *Frontiers in Psychology*.
   2019;10:2677.

2. American Foundation for Suicide Prevention. *After a Suicide: A Toolkit for Schools*,
   2nd ed. Waltham, MA: Education Development Center; 2018. Retrieved 6/24/22.
   https://afsp.org/after-a-suicide-a-toolkit-for-schools.

3. Erbacher TA, Singer JB, Poland S. *Suicide in Schools: A Practitioner's Guide to
   Multi-Level Prevention, Assessment, Intervention, and Postvention.* New York:
   Routledge; 2014.

4. Abrutyn S, Mueller AS. Are Suicidal Behaviors Contagious? Using Longitudinal Data
   to Examine Suicide Suggestion. *American Sociological Review*. 2014;79(2):211–227.

5. American Foundation for Suicide Prevention. State Laws: Suicide Prevention in
   Schools (K-12). 2020. Retrieved 4/26/22. https://www.datocms-assets.com/12810/
   1602535612-k-1602535612-schools-issue-brief-1602535610-1602535612-1602535
   620.pdf.

6. American Foundation for Suicide Prevention. *After a Suicide: A Toolkit for Schools*,
   1st ed. 2011.

7. Diefendorf S, Van Norden S, Abrutyn S, Mueller AS. Understanding Suicide
   Bereavement, Contagion, and the Importance of Thoughtful Postvention in Schools.
   In: Ackerman JP, Horowitz LM, eds. *Youth Suicide Prevention and Intervention*.
   New York: Springer; 2022:51–60.

8. Williams DY, Wexler L, Mueller AS. Suicide Postvention in Schools: What Evidence
   Supports Our Current National Recommendations? *School Social Work Journal*.
   2022;46(3):23–69.

9. Singer JB, Erbacher TA, Rosen P. School-Based Suicide Prevention: A Framework
   for Evidence-Based Practice. *School Mental Health*. 2019;11(1):54–71.

10. Hallett T. The Myth Incarnate: Recoupling Processes, Turmoil, and Inhabited Institutions in an Urban Elementary School. *American Sociological Review.* 2010;75:52–74.

11. Marsh I. *Suicide: Foucault, History and Truth.* Cambridge, UK: Cambridge University Press; 2010.

12. Mueller AS, Abrutyn S. Suicidal Disclosures Among Friends: Using Social Network Data to Understand Suicide Contagion. *Journal of Health and Social Behavior.* 2015;56(1):131–148.

13. Mueller AS. Does the Media Matter to Suicide? Examining the Social Dynamics Surrounding Media Reporting on Suicide in a Suicide-Prone Community. *Social Science and Medicine.* 2017;180:152–159.

14. O'Connor R. *When It Is Darkest: Why People Die by Suicide and What We Can Do to Prevent It.* New York: Random House; 2021.

6

SAFER MEMORIALIZATION

Every year, in the fall, around the United States, people who have lost loved ones to suicide gather for a ritual "Out of Darkness Walk" hosted by local chapters of the American Foundation for Suicide Prevention. Walkers don colored beads to indicate why they are there—purple for the loss of a friend or relative; white for the loss of a child; teal if you support someone who struggles with suicidality; blue for supporting the cause of suicide prevention. The events aim to put a face to suicide, to bring suicide out of the shadows and demand—by literally stopping traffic through towns and cities—attention be paid to the pain and suffering that this public health crisis is wreaking on the nation.

In Poplar Grove's countywide Out of Darkness Walk, the event is in equal parts a memorial ritual for loved ones lost and a passionate campaign to build awareness about suicide and fight mental health stigma. The mourning and activism mingle somewhat awkwardly: some people stand away from the crowd, in quiet groups marked by somber faces, while others seem to treat the march as a reunion—joyfully greeting friends they haven't seen in a while. Still, the truth that draws them there is never far from the surface. They are parents, children, siblings, friends, and significant others of people who have died by suicide. They are survivors enduring a pain often described as unimaginable for anyone who hasn't experienced it. Even in seemingly happy crowds, the pain is always there.

It is startling to look around and see all the teams walking in memory of Poplar Grove kids. Many of the teams are quite large, with teen and adult walkers wearing matching t-shirts, bracelets saying "Forever Remember," memorabilia inspired by their loved one's favorite color or motto, and nods to the personalities of those they've lost. It's a stark visual reminder of just how many people have been impacted by suicide in Poplar Grove.

Anna stands wearing beads of teal and blue, waiting to begin the walk with the group honoring Aria. A young girl she recognizes as Aria's little sister runs past and flings herself, sobbing, into her father's arms. Roughly 40 kids, teens, and parents milling about near Anna are swept up in the girl's grief, crumpling as Aria's sister cries. Aria's father holds his surviving daughter quietly. He's a rock, but Anna can see how hard it is for him to hold it all together—to hold his little girl up, to hold his family up, to hold his community up.

While schools are one of the most important institutions for suicide postvention, they are far from the only place where communities gather to process suicide losses and convey messages, deliberately or inadvertently, about mental health, grief, and suicide. Mourning rituals like funerals and memorial services are designed to help bond surviving community members together, to allow social support to flow to those in need, to help make sense of the loss of a cherished individual, and at times, to help ensure that the community does not fall apart when tragedy strikes.[1,2] These powerful rituals can strengthen our collective bonds by affirming that community members matter to each other, that the loss of one affects all. They also help solidify the memory of a particular event into a shared story—a collective memory—about what happened, who was impacted, how the community healed, and how they reaffirmed their faith in each other through a collective response.[3] In a word, mourning rituals both create and sustain a shared cultural memory that anchors community members to a collective idenity.[4] They have the potential to impart important messages: you are not alone; you matter; your community cares.

But when it comes to suicide postvention, scholars and clinicians have serious concerns about how we mass memorialize people who have died by suicide. There are two main reasons for their concerns. First, if we mourn suicide losses differently than other deaths, we could stigmatize people who have died by suicide, conveying to their community that they mattered less than their peers. For instance, if a church has a moment of silence during Sunday services in honor of a youth who died from cancer, but does not do the same for a youth who died by suicide, that can communicate that certain lives and deaths are more worthy of recognition than others.[5] This can cause terrible pain for bereaved friends and family. Fortunately, this is not a particular concern in Poplar Grove, where community groups were quick to recognize the pain of bereaved individuals and to honor the memory of any youth who died prematurely, regardless of cause, though the cause of death—suicide—may not be openly discussed.

A second concern with memorialization is far more relevant to Poplar Grove: that massive, well-attended memorials where everyone discusses the amazing person who died can provide opportunities for the social comparison of grieving and the social contagion of emotions like grief and fear. These events can also inadvertently glorify or romanticize suicide as an option, sending confusing messages about suicide (particularly when not combined with effective postvention or prevention strategies). Any of these outcomes, experts suggest, may render a community more vulnerable to suicide clusters.[6]

Given these concerns, to fully understand the making of the suicide problem in Poplar Grove we must ask: How did Poplar Grove's collective mourning rituals contribute to the experience of suicide in the community? Did they promote healing and provide support? Or were they another place where youth encountered silence, stigma, and confusing messages about what it means to die by suicide? Examining how kids experienced mourning rituals and listening to what messages they took away from them is critical to understanding how youth make sense of suicide and how their understanding can shift in response to the personal experience of suicide loss. In so doing, we also hope to provide insights into how we can honor the memories of the loved ones we have lost to suicide while also protecting the vulnerable grieving kids and families left behind—the survivors of suicide.

6.1 THE COMMUNITY GATHERS

In Poplar Grove, the dense social networks that draw community members into each other's lives also draw them together in the wake of tragedy. This is quite evident through attendance at the funerals, vigils, and memorial services of youth who died by suicide. In Poplar Grove, these mourning rituals are well attended, particularly when the youth who died was an ideal-typical kid or when their family is deeply integrated into the community. For example, Aria's memorial service was described, by her parents and her friends, as including "thousands" of people. Similarly, when Anna asked Beth and her (young adult) friends what it was like to go to memorial services, Beth—referencing Michelle's service—retorted, "Crowded." Gwen added:

> I remember walking in [to Michelle's service], and the whole cheerleading team was in their uniform on the floor, in each other's arms crying. I remember a big chunk of the soccer team basically doing the same thing. I remember there were, like, parents of her friends, there were, like, neighbors. Like, literally, like, if you knew Michelle at all, I feel like you were there. Like the whole funeral home . . . they opened up all the rooms . . . [T]he line was out the door.

Molly and Vanessa confirmed that Michelle's memorial was so "crowded" that some people had to stand in the hallway for the service. Brian's service was described as having hundreds in attendance, as was Quinn's. "There were so many people," Leah said, recalling Quinn's memorial service. "People were standing in the aisles," her best friend Kaitlyn chimed in, "It was literally our community."

It is not surprising that the memorial services tended to be crowded. In a community defined by an ethos of support and connectedness, people wanted to show up and be there for those who were grieving. And for many family members, the high attendance really did help them feel supported in an overwhelming moment of grief. Lauren's mother Sandra said, with gratitude, "At her funeral . . . it was standing room only.

Hundreds of hundreds of hundreds of people come up to me saying, 'Oh, I knew Lauren, I'm from Vollentine,' which is 35 minutes away. Or, 'Hey, I know Lauren!' I'm like, 'How did she know all these people?!'"

But there were other consequences of the strong sense of community when it came to mourning in Poplar Grove. People's grief at the memorial services was intense. "I remember I was crying really loudly," Beth shared, reflecting on how she felt at Michelle's memorial service during a group conversation. "It was really emotional. I remember one of my counselors in my youth group was behind me, and she put her hand on my shoulder to calm me down." And youth noticed what they called "weird waves" of emotion that would pass through the crowd of kids, "where it's like everyone feels sad at the same time." There were also moments of collective calm: "Like everyone was like, 'let's, like, be okay for, like, 15 minutes right now.' Obviously it's not like you're required to be on the same wavelength," Beth explained, "But, like, I don't know."

"It's nice," Molly chimed in, about feeling that emotional synchronicity. "It's like a tight-knit community," Elisha said, and while the waves of emotions were intense, they also felt "nice." Being tied together in grief reaffirmed the sense of Poplar Grove being a tightly interconnected community. No one was grieving alone. "I feel like that's always good," Elisha shared. Indeed, many youth (and adults) appreciated the public outpourings of love and the copious attention that flowed out of funerals. Leah felt "kinda happy" that "hundreds" came to Quinn's funeral, and mentioned looking around and seeing faces of people she remembered Quinn talking about "all the time." It made her think, "Oh my God, [Quinn would] be so excited to know that so-and-so was here.'"

It can be positive to experience outpourings of love and other emotions that help youth know they're not alone. There's nothing quite like the reassuring hand on your shoulder that says your grief is witnessed. Still, there were downsides to the intense displays of emotion at Poplar Grove suicide memorials. The very ties that drew so many people to memorial services, regardless of how close they were to the grieving family, also exposed them to the intense grief of others, which in turn sometimes intensified their own grief experience. "I don't get why [Isla is] this upset,"

Krista confessed, thinking back on a girl she went to church with who was extremely distraught at Michelle's memorial service: "She didn't even know [Michelle], so her brokenness [in the wake of Michelle's death] . . . [I'm just] not understanding why they are reacting in this way." Almost every youth we spoke to who was highly impacted by suicide shared a story about being upset, or mad, or frustrated by other youth attendees who they perceived were grieving too much or in ways that did not align with how close they seemed to be to the memorialized youth during their life.

Many of these concerns centered on teens engaging in what young Poplar Grovians sometimes labeled "attention-seeking" behaviors. For Luke, Kennedy's funeral was upsetting more because of the people he was exposed to than his own raw emotions at the sudden death of a life-long friend. "I ended up reacting more to just the people around me" than to Kennedy's death, at least initially, Luke shared, "sort of like judging and hating them [for it] because it was just annoying." He was particularly angry that he was able to "hold [him]self together in public without making a big show [when] people who, like, had two classes with her and they're like, 'Oh, Kennedy!'" He mimicked their sobbing. "They . . . turned it into, like, a 'me' thing. You know?" Jack agreed: he'd largely wanted to be left alone to grieve in the privacy of his tight-knit group of friends or with Kennedy's family, but the memorial services ended up being a mixed bag for him. Jack recalled:

It was good for me to talk at [her formal memorial service]. I don't know if it was cathartic, but I guess it was nice to have something to say. And everyone was massively supportive. But at the same time . . . it felt like a lot of people were trying to piggyback on this and get attention really. . . . [P]eople were clamoring to be the one who was affected by it. There's no soft way to say it. Like, there were girls who were getting tattoos with her name on it. And I remember another high school guy who—suddenly he just wanted to tell everyone how close he [was to Kennedy] . . . I mean, it's also just high school kids, but that aspect of [the memorial service], and coming together so everyone can feel sorry for themselves? I think it bothered me.

Jack understood part of what happened at Kennedy's memorial service could be chalked up to high schoolers being high schoolers, yet the amplification of grieving that he witnessed disturbed him.

Other kids who lost other friends noticed the same thing. June felt angry at the other kids who showed up at Michelle's memorial service. "I was just like, 'You didn't really know her, and you're acting like you're really upset,'" June scoffed. "To me, I was just, like, angry because I was just like, 'You're, like, making this, you just want to *feed* off of something.'"

Same thing at Quinn's memorial. "I have this one really close friend who knew Quinn from elementary school," Shannon began with a frown. "Right when Quinn died, [my friend] she'd just tell people, 'Oh, my mom works with her mom—I can't believe this happened!' and I'm like 'What?! That connection is so irrelevant right now! Like, it literally means nothing!!'" For Shannon, the friend was just making the story about herself, rather than about Quinn, her family, and her highly impacted friends.

6.2 THE COMPLEXITIES OF COLLECTIVE MOURNING

We did not feel it was appropriate for us to attend any of these memorial services or vigils ourselves, so we cannot provide an observational account. However, we can leverage our knowledge of the town, our understanding of grief in adolescence and adolescent development, and our conversations with youth both highly and tangentially impacted by a peer's death to offer some context to the so-called attention-seeking behavior so many of our interlocutors found upsetting.

First, because of the tight-knit social networks and strong community identity in Poplar Grove, what happened to one person seemed to matter to many more community members than might be the case in a larger, more heterogeneous city. Here, where students shared a school, a neighborhood, or a faith community, each suicide loss "gripped our town" (to quote Shannon), absorbing everyone into the tragedy.

"It was a big freaking thing that happened," Denise said of her best friend Julia's death. And while Denise, like Luke, Jack, Shannon, and others, could be angry about what she saw as the attention-seeking, over-wrought grief performances of kids who barely knew the deceased, she also acknowledged that "just because they weren't as close as I was to the situation . . . and just because they were more vocal about what was going on with them, who's to say that that's not a[n appropriate] way of dealing with it? It was a big freaking thing," she repeated, "and the fallout was different for everyone."

Ander, who was not close to any decedents, though he had been school and classmates with some, captured this perfectly:

It's just people you have these interactions with and you know so personally—and impersonally sometimes . . . But it *feels* so personal once they are gone, because you remember all those times you did interact with them on a personal level and they become more real or more meaningful . . . you experience that hurt . . . and then you empathize with people they did know closely. *Cool* is not the word to use to describe this, but I'm proud of the community in Poplar Grove for kind of the way we've responded. Definitely [we] could do things better, maybe we should have done things better, but the fact that we did respond—it's cool to see that when one person loses their life in the community, it's not like they're an island. The whole community responds. So, hundreds of people have responded to five, six, or seven, ten people [whose deaths] have caused a huge ripple effect.

Isla's grief, which so perplexed Krista, becomes more understandable when we contextualize it within Poplar Grove's strong sense of community. These mourning rituals were intensely emotional. Youth witnessed many people that they knew, people who were like them, grieving intensely. Isla, for instance, almost certainly saw Beth's uncontrolled sobs and almost certainly identified with Beth, as she did with Michelle. These young women had so much in common—they shared their school, a religious youth group, and a community. They are Poplar Grove.

It is possible then that these large memorials, gathering people who shared a strong social identity and who often knew each other, facilitated the social contagion of mourning. Remember the wave of grief Anna saw cascade through the crowd at the Out of Darkness Walk—when one person started to cry, they all broke down. Waves like these almost certainly washed over Isla, just as they did Beth, Krista, and others. A broad body of research has identified this propensity for emotions to spread through crowds.[7] This contagion of emotions is not necessarily a bad thing. Witnessing grief allows us to imagine, and almost even experience, how others might feel, increasing empathy, compassion, and the sense of a shared experience.[8] But it's also not necessarily a good thing. The same process, of course, can raise the number of people who are grieving or intensify people's experience of grief; some youth may not have felt such intense grief without the exposure to others at the memorial services, which made other's pain more personal. Considered this way, we can reimagine Isla's response to Michelle's death: neither strange nor overwrought, Isla's intense reaction becomes, from this perspective, understandable, and possibly even expected.

None of us is privileged to know the entire history of others' relationships or the complexities of their grief. Some kids who, to peers, seemed like attention-seekers may have had long-lapsed but still meaningful to them childhood friendships with the person who died. Others may have recently lost someone else they cared about to suicide—perhaps someone who didn't attend Poplar Grove High School or even live in Poplar Grove. For them, grief over the loss of their peer may blend with grief over loss of their loved one, but others wouldn't necessarily know that. For other kids, their grieving can be inflected by emotions like guilt or anger, which make it hard to process a sudden and tragic loss upending their high school and their community. Perhaps they have regrets, perhaps they weren't the kindest to the person who died, and they are reckoning with that. Indeed, in our conversations with different young Poplar Grovians, we found examples of all of the above that help explain why some youth were considered surprisingly impacted by a peer's death.

That said, an understandable pattern of exaggerated public reactions to loss remains a cause for concern. When youth report that they have lost a friend to suicide or a friend has attempted suicide, they are, on average, more likely to develop suicidal thoughts or attempt suicide themselves, even if we hold other risk and protective factors for suicide constant.[9,10] This means that exposure to a peer's suicide attempt or death actually increases a teen's risk of experiencing suicidality, particularly when their community is marked by mental health stigma, as in Poplar Grove, and lacks strong postvention practices. Given that Poplar Grove has experienced recurring suicide clusters and, as reported to us by local mental, physical, and public health professionals, that almost *every* suicide death in Poplar Grove was followed by multiple other suicide attempts if not deaths, the spread of intense grief throughout the town's young people— possibly heightening their sense of connection with the deceased—is a very real and concerning situation. It's even potentially dangerous.

6.3 ROMANTIZING SUICIDE

Memorials for youth who have died by suicide also have the potential to romanticize suicide as an option for others. The idea is that mass mourning can somehow make suicide seem like a way to achieve prominence or gain the attention youth often crave. While the guidelines for suicide postvention often caution against romanticizing suicide, they provide no examples of what romanticization looks like or what harm it might do.

In Poplar Grove, our own observations and those of community members offered some romanticizing red flags. When "the whole village" shows up for a funeral, for instance, youth may see that substantial attention from peers and adults, attention which may seem scarce in life, can be abundant in death. Parents Frank and Patricia worried along these lines:

PATRICIA: It does take a village to prevent [suicide], but then the village shows up for the funeral . . . and it's like—

FRANK: [interjecting] Where were you before?

PATRICIA: I mean, for people who are already in that zone [thinking about suicide], it's like "Look at all these people!" . . . when [before their peer died], nobody was aware that anything was going on with this kid. And then the village shows up at the end, and it's like . . . it sends completely the wrong message.

Helen, a community mental health worker, said similarly: "I think Michelle's death couldn't be more glorified . . . I mean, if you want attention, if you want to be the *star of the town* for a short period of time, 'Why don't you kill yourself?' . . . Michelle got [that attention], you know?"

We found evidence that at least some youth who died by suicide had been aware that suicide raises one's profile, as it were. Many of the Poplar Grove youth who died by suicide had either attended huge memorials or were aware of the massive attendance at peers' funerals. In Lauren's case, this had even come up in conversation with her mother, Sandra. "I remember once, a few years ago" Sandra recounted, "I remember Lauren once just telling me, 'Mom, if I ever died, I would have so many friends come to my funeral,' because she and I were having a battle about friends or something. And I was like, 'No, Lauren, you wouldn't, because it would be closed and I wouldn't let any of your friends in!'" While that didn't happen—Sandra welcomed Lauren's friends to her funeral—this memory gave Sandra pause. When we discussed Lauren's memorial service with Sandra, she first shared how wonderful the outpouring of support made her feel. But she also noted feeling concerned about all the kids who were in attendance—did it harm them? At her own daughter's funeral, Sandra went around, actively trying to prevent other kids from tattooing Lauren's death date on their forearms and to connect grieving kids to care.

Lily confirmed that kids did imagine and talk about what it would be like if they died—comments that returned to the pressures of the Poplar Grove ideal. As she said, "A lot of people think 'What would people think if I [died by suicide]?" To Lily, though, these musings were normal. She continued:

I feel like everybody does that, almost in any place. Like, "Oh what would happen if I died? What will people say?" Not just because you want people to remember you like that and you want to be able to be there for your funeral or something. It's more like, "What would people think? Would they look at my GPA? Would they look at all of the things that I did well, instead of the things that I didn't do?"

Before her death, Aria journaled about her funeral. She wrote about her curiosity—how would friends react "to hearing the news" of her death "or going to the funeral"? This line of thinking wasn't always saturated with positive emotions. "I start to bawl," Aria wrote in one passage. Her friends, she thought, "don't deserve to be hurt by me like that." But she was also aware of the power of her death. She wrote, for example, on the day of her death, that the date "is always going to be remembered. The day that will be on my tombstone, the date on the funeral program, the date that will haunt at least a dozen people for a life time." She wasn't wrong. It's hard not to think about Aria as the date of her death rolls around, year after year, even for those of us who never had the pleasure of knowing her in life.

At funerals and memorials, youth think about death. They pick up both tacit and explicit messages about death. And at times, youth feel that the messages "glamorize" suicide. Returning to Luke's anger at Kennedy's memorial service, we can see that the reaction was partially driven by what he felt was his peers' attention-seeking behavior, but it was also related to what people were saying about Kennedy. "The vibe was kind of like, 'She had it figured out.'" In this moment, Luke was sharing intense anger; he was very mad at Kennedy for what he saw as her choice to die. His words may be hard for some to read. His voice rose:

[P]eople were telling stories about her, and like . . . , "Oh, yeah. Let's remember the *good*." And I felt like, at times, I was like, "Am I the only one that, like, hates her guts and thinks she's a piece of shit [for what she did]?" You know? . . . I mean, there were a couple who were on the same page with me [like, let's not glorify her choice], but you know, like, her one really good friend was Francesca, that I dated for a little bit. Yeah. She just, like, totally thought Kennedy had it figured out. Kind of turned her into a martyr.

While Luke didn't truly hate Kennedy, he hated what she did to him, to her friends, and especially, to her family. He hated that no one talked about the harm she caused by her death.

Youth consistently told us that the tendency to focus on the "good" was a theme across memorial services. Adults were no less aware. Diane, a mom whose daughter lost a friend to suicide, was furious after attending the funeral. "She was sick. People don't just kill themselves. They don't just wake up and have a bad day. If you are in that place, it's sickness. It's mental sickness," she insisted. "Why don't we just *say* that at these [memorial gatherings]?! [But no.] Instead we say 'She was such a good athlete, she was a beautiful girl.'" While Diane's language is a bit stigmatizing, her point is that focusing on only the good and not also talking about the girl's struggle was not necessarily helpful for the students bearing witness to her death and memorial.

As a result, the messages that many of young Poplar Grovians took away from the majority of the memorial services was that the person who died was placed on a "pedestal." "Like with Michelle," Lily shared, "We think of her as so high up and everything. No one really talks about 'Oh, she [killed herself.].'" Hannah continued the conversation, concurring:

HANNAH: It's glamorized. How she died.

LILY: Yeah.

HANNAH: She's put on a pedestal.

MADISON: It's like, no one talks about the fact that she did take her life. But she didn't talk about it to anyone, so nobody knew. And we don't talk about the fact that that did happen, and we still don't know. I admit, I guess it's not public information, but we don't know what was wrong. Like, why was she sad?

Ben quietly answered Madison's sincere question: "She had a diagnosed mental illness. She was clinically depressed."

That information triggered Hannah to share of Michelle: "She was about to go back into treatment, I think . . . she just wanted to take care of her grades before she went back into treatment, and she just couldn't make

[it]. . . . [T]hat's what I've been told. . . . I'm not close to the family, but if that's true, that's tragic." Madison protested: "But nobody remembers that!" Even if mental illness and treatment were part of Michelle's story, it was not the main message evoked by her funeral. Instead, "nobody remembers why" Michelle died by suicide, Madison declared.

Hannah picked the conversation back up on the idea of the memorial focusing on how wonderful Michelle was:

HANNAH: She's put on a pedestal. I'm not saying she's a bad person, 'cause I'm sure that she was an amazing person. But it's become, like, everybody loves Michelle, and I think if you were going through a hard time and you looked at that, you'd be like, "I could just end this, and everybody would love me, and I wouldn't have any more problems." 'Cause instead of using it as "This is what could happen," it's like, "Oh, we miss her so much. She was such a good person."

MADISON: It's like, "That *can* happen. That's what I want to do."

HANNAH: It's like, "That won't happen again. That was a freak accident." It's just glamorized . . . extremely. It's not blaming the family, because I know they're going through a really hard time emotionally, but it's just like, the whole town. They're trying to be loving and understanding, but it's just a bad example.

Luke felt the same about all the positive attention showered on Kennedy: "I honestly think that [the positive attention] had a lot to do with you know, a lot of these attempted suicides [that followed Kennedy's death]. A lot of these were like cries for attention, in my opinion, and I think they saw how much attention she got. She got so much attention. She was just turned into, like, a total martyr."

These kids have a lot to teach us—and Poplar Grove—about the dangers of what's *not* said, particularly in the context of massive memorial services. Memories, explanations, and meanings are collectively constructed at these events. Because, as we explored in earlier chapters, having a mental health problem is positioned here as something contrary to being a "good" kid, Poplar Grove's memorial services made little space to discuss mental health or suicide. Kids even felt what sociologists call a normative pressure to keep the conversation positive like those around them were doing—to "not trash talk the dead kid," as it were. Where suicide was stigmatized as an expression of mental illness, simply naming the cause of death could be seen as calling the deceased a "bad" person.

The rules of positivity and silence can leave kids completely confused. Where is their seemingly perfect classmate now? Gone by suicide. But why? And could it happen again?

6.4 ADULTS VERSUS KIDS

Amelia acknowledged that she wasn't as impacted by the suicide losses in Poplar Grove as other kids were. She was friendly with Michelle—they sat together in class—but they weren't close friends. And she only knew Mark through school extracurricular activities. When we asked about attending memorial services, her main emotion was frustration. "I wanted there to be more support, more rallying," she shared. "If I had a friend who completed suicide, then I would be rallying. I would be spreading the awareness and really trying to help people." Amelia tried to do this following her classmate's suicide death. "They decided that it was disrespectful," though, she said with evident annoyance. "I understand that the family has to grieve, but I guess I'm just different from them in a way where, when something bad happens, I don't like to just hold it inside. . . . I'm the kind of person that wants to change it, and make it better. So, it was very *very* frustrating."

Amelia and her peers started an online group called Teens Against Suicide. "But of course, it got shut down, because they decided it was disrespectful to the girl's family," she explained. "They decided that [the online group] was going to create the 'ripple effect,' and more kids were going to commit suicide, and cut themselves, and they didn't let us do any kind of memorial services either [outside of the funeral]."

"They," unnamed and ominous, stood in for a generalized Poplar Grove adult in Amelia's comments. And indeed, we had also experienced and heard frequent references to "their" fear of possibly instigating a suicide cluster. Even though staying silent about suicide is not an element of safe suicide postvention, this overarching fear seemed to encourage silence, even suppression, in Poplar Grove.

Her active pursuit of suicide information led Amelia to gatherings of adults following losses. "I went to this one thing at Willow Creek Church" after Michelle's suicide, she remembered, "where it was like, 'What should parents do when there is a suicide in the community?' They were like, 'We have to keep it very *quiet*, and very *hushed*.' And 'We want to make sure that [youth and parents] understand, but we also don't want to create the ripple effect.'" It's likely the message was more involved, but this is what Amelia took away from the experience. It impacted her deeply:

> I feel like they're so scared of that ripple effect that they're confusing the rest of us. I want to be able to talk about [suicide]! I want to be able to have it out in the open! Because it clears a lot of the confusion, and it gives you closure. But they are so scared that there are going to be kids that fall through the cracks, that they leave the rest of us kind of . . . in the dark. And that's what happened with Mark. They left us completely in the dark, and I still don't have a closure about [his death].

Anna prompted Amelia, noting that she'd mentioned "you want *information*—*" At this, Amelia murmured in agreement. "—so that *you* know what to do. And, if there's no conversation, I imagine that also—"

Amelia interrupted, "Yeah. After Mark died, they didn't do anything about teaching us what to look for. They didn't even say that it was a suicide. I had to hear that it was a suicide from one of his friends. They just said it was a *death*. They didn't say it was a suicide."

"And would you say that . . . you know," Anna began haltingly. "So, it sounds like the adult community tried to shut down the conversation about Michelle. But would you say that the adolescent community just kept talking?"

Again, Amelia confirmed: "Mmhmm."

"So, it didn't really shut down anything, it just shut the official conversation? Or the public conversation, so it was more private?

Yes, the girl nodded. "It was more private. It was more 'kept to the kids.'"

Ultimately, Amelia's verdict about suicide prevention and postvention in Poplar Grove was that "it feels very 'adult versus teenager.'" As in the previous chapter, Amelia echoed the theme that, in the wake of a suicide, adults weren't people youth could rely on. Generally, kids felt that adults wanted to sweep the repeated suicides under the rug, and that they didn't really understand how scary it was for kids to see their peers taking their own lives, to grow up with suicide as a recurring and defining experience. Interestingly, this theme was also present in our conversations with the mental health workers in the community, who critiqued the silence they perceived among parents and other Poplar Grove adults. "I'm really concerned," Douglas, a mental health worker, shared. "I would take a good guess that most parents don't have 'the suicide conversation' with their child."

That was Molly's experience. As we learned in the previous chapter, Molly was directly impacted by the death of Michelle, yet she felt her parents failed to understand what she was going through. "I was so angry at my parents for never doing anything and never talking to me about [Michelle's death]. I just couldn't believe that," Molly shared. "I think things would've been different if [my dad] had been in town [for Michelle's funeral]. I think he would've understood the gravity of the situation a little more."

Likewise, a parent told us it took a fight with her daughter to understand the depth of her grief. Diane, the mother, shared that her daughter came to her crying with the news that her friend had died by suicide. Sadly, Diane remembered, her first response was to say, "She was not your best friend." Diane shared, "That's an odd thing to say, [I realize now]. I look back on that and realize it was very hurtful." Her daughter was understandably furious.

For Madison, the struggle to talk with her mom about what she was going through seemed stymied by her mother's own inability to process.

Her mom didn't "know how to deal with" the fact that her friend had died by suicide, she figured. Madison explained:

> Like last week, we were driving somewhere and [I mentioned it was four years since Mark died] . . . and she goes off on a little rant, like . . . "Don't you wish he didn't kill himself?" Blah blah blah . . . and I'm like, "MOM STOP." . . . She cares. She wants me to be okay, but then, she hasn't, like, dealt with this before, so she doesn't know how to deal with it. Which is a problem for her . . . she won't know how to deal with this, and she goes into her angry moment."

Certainly, supporting children through grief and loss is extremely difficult for parents. "It got to be a lot for me," Diane admitted. We get it. The situation was absolutely terrifying for Diane: "My daughter would fall apart. She would be hysterical. You know things would be good, and then hysterical." Years after the fact, Diane's interview was peppered with tears and anger. Parents want to keep their kids safe and provide them with the ideal childhood. Quite frankly, that does not include exposure to suicide. Diane didn't sign up for life in Poplar Grove expecting that she'd weather repeated calls to alert her or her children that yet another youth was dead by suicide, or to find herself learning how to support youth through grief and tragedy. It's difficult to face these incidents as it is, and it can be harder yet for adults to pull themselves together and, without training, say helpful, supportive things that get through to the children in their lives. And if the first words an adult utters to a kid are hurtful or "wrong," they're so hard to take back. Adults seemed understandably angry, too; just as kids expected adults to communicate and take charge, adults felt the school and the community should be leading postvention. Surely experts should be brought in. "There was no collective sense of, 'This is what we should do. These are experts in the field. They deal with this all the time,'" Denise, a young adult and suicide loss survivor, said. She couldn't think of any adults who, drawing on scientific and clinical evidence, came in and, authoritatively, took charge to ensure students were supported with appropriate suicide postvention. Kids and parents alike experienced additional suffering because of this lack.

Naturally, kids simply talked about suicide amongst themselves. Some snuck off to hold midnight vigils in graveyards, hiding where they went and what they were doing. They tried to figure out how to keep each other safe and keep the memory of their friends alive. They did not necessarily know how to talk about suicide without romanticizing it. They didn't know how to address their peers' intense grief or "attention-seeking"—what we might more fruitfully call *help-craving* behaviors. They were simply compelled to figure out what was killing kids. And their experiences with suicide were so intense that silence just wasn't going to work for kids.

6.5 COULD WE BE NEXT?

One consequence of the recurring suicides and recurring silences was that kids became skittish, wary that tragedy was around every corner. Could their stressed-out best friend be next? Could *they* be next?

Teenager Hannah's account was visceral:

[The repeating suicides are] giving me a little bit of—not really anxiety, but *anxiety*. Because you don't know who it could be. Like, if it could be *these people* that didn't seem like they're having issues, then how do you know, if your friend is having a bad day, that they're not thinking about committing suicide? You know what I mean? So, I know I'm always worried about that. And that stresses me out, because I would have never have guessed that that would have happened. So how do I know that it's not going to happen again, to somebody that I know really closely? You can only control yourself. You can be really kind, and you can do all these things, but you still don't know how a person is really feeling.

Hannah, explaining the deaths of these popular peers as due to academic and social pressure, grew vigilant toward her own friends' well-being. When other kids—admired kids with no publicly visible signs of distress—take their own lives, it raises troubling questions for their fellow youth. It's all compounded when adults fail to provide factual information that explains the complexity and relative rarity of suicide, the role of psychological pain, and that some people choose to hide their psychological pain from the public—all conversations that are, in fact, possible and perfectly compatible with respecting families' wishes and incorporating up-to-date best practices.

After Michelle's death, "a lot of the kids were just like, 'Oh my gosh, that's gonna be us!' " Natalie explained. " 'We're all gonna stress out and lose it.' Even if your life is great, you can still snap one day." But in general, people *don't* just snap and take their lives. Many suicide attempts are described as "impulsive," though research (including our own community-based work) suggests the links between youth, impulsivity, and suicide are quite nuanced. For instance, youth with impulsive personality traits may, on average, be more vulnerable to thinking about and attempting suicide,[11] yet there isn't a difference in the impulsivity between those youth who just think about suicide and those who attempt or complete suicide.[12,13] This suggests that possessing impulsive personality traits may render youth less able to cope with the negative events and emotions the world throws at them, but it doesn't necessarily mean that impulsivity plays a major role in a teen escalating from suicidal thoughts to a suicide attempt or death.

Researchers further report that youths' reactions to how they feel, particularly to negative emotions—what is sometimes called their more- or less-developed emotional regulation skills—are at least as key to their vulnerability to thinking about and, for girls, attempting suicide.[14] Equally important, we know that even if higher impulsivity increases the risk of suicidality, it is very possible to intervene in that pathway by building youth's emotional regulation skills and teaching them early warning signs so they understand when to ask for and how to get help. Kids like Natalie have lots of options to ensure they do not just "snap" and die by suicide. Making sure that they know this—that they understand their own ability to control their psychological futures—is crucial to suicide prevention.

To a large extent, however, that education wasn't happening for Poplar Grove kids. Instead, for at least some kids, exposure to recurring suicides combined with the shower of attention that fell on the kids who had died by suicide and the lack of effective postvention meant that suicide seemed like a possible solution to their problems. "I've wanted to get away from having all these problems," Becca shared. "Seeing all these other people go through all these problems, their answer is suicide, so why can't my answer be suicide?" Madison shared a similar sentiment, which we also heard in an earlier chapter:

> Like, four years [after Mark's death] . . . I would think like, "Mark had so many issues of his own, and now he doesn't have them anymore." Like, how great would that be? To not have to, like, go through your life thinking about every little thing that you do. . . . So, it's just kind of like, "*What a great idea. Like, you don't have to, like, deal with any of your problems anymore. Like, you could just* be." [emphasis added]

For Becca and Madison, these are just thoughts—sometimes comforting thoughts that help them feel a sense of control. Still, such thoughts can make suicide more accessible for teenagers, more imaginable, more applicable to their own lives. A large body of research confirms that an individual's beliefs about suicide's acceptability or reasonableness as an action heighten their risk for and atrophy barriers to future suicidality.[15,16] Additionally, the more youth identify themselves with death, the more vulnerable they are to suicidality.[17]

Taken together, the research says that Becca and Madison's beliefs about suicide as a possible solution to their own problems is concerning. Should their psychological pain ever get to a point that it overwhelms their ability to cope, their experiences may make them more vulnerable than if they had had different experiences with suicide, postvention, and memorialization.

6.6 THE BENEFITS OF GATHERING IN GRIEF, SAFELY

One of the challenging things in talking and writing about memorialization is that so much is out of our control. It's very difficult to tell a grieving family how to manage their child's memorial. We aren't even sure we would recommend that—it feels too disrespectful to the family. Collective grieving rituals can also be healing for people who are suffering, including youth. Excluding some youth from memorial services may not be a great idea. At the same time, we are fairly convinced that large, well-attended memorials have unintended negative mental health consequences.

We have, in our years of careful community research, notice two powerful ways to make memorials safer and help them play a positive role in suicide prevention. The first is to talk openly about suicide at the memorial; the second is to talk openly about the pain of grieving. Together, the two seem to aid in *social inoculation* of youth against suicide.

6.6.1 Talk Openly About Suicide

One memorial service and one family stood apart from the standard Poplar Grove pattern of focusing on the good, rather than speaking about how and why a youth died. From the very beginning, Aria's parents were open about the fact that their daughter had died by suicide. They spoke about what was, in all likelihood, Aria's undiagnosed mental illness (specifically, they believed, bipolar disorder). They talked passionately about ending the stigma and silence around mental illness and suicide. And they even role-modeled open conversation by talking personally about mental illness and help-seeking in intimate community spaces, on local and national news, and even during Aria's memorial service. "Aria shone bright as a diamond on the outside," read the memorial message Aria's parents shared with us following the service, "but there was a darkness inside her that we didn't see. Her life was full. But the darkness was overwhelming. We didn't know she was struggling with depression."

As they adopted their new role as advocates for suicide prevention, Aria's parents normalized getting help, in part by sharing what it was like for Aria's father to live with his mental illness. All about ending the stigma, Josie declared, "[Mental illness] is like a disease, like cancer or diabetes. It's something that—probably more comparable to diabetes, because it's something you just have to live with. And there is no shame in having to take insulin." They helped organize suicide prevention efforts at events, like rock concerts, that drew kids and parents, with booths hosted by county suicide prevention organizations (e.g., the local mental health crisis center). They asked questions of local suicide prevention experts (including us) on how to hone their message and their activities to best reach kids and prevent suicide. All this made it feel easier, maybe even cool, for youth to learn about suicide prevention.

Will and Josie allowed people to publicly witness their pain, their enduring love for Aria, and their firm stance that suicide and mental illness are *not* shameful. Period. Friendly and easy to admire, the couple's honesty could be disarming. In his remarks at the memorial, Will said, "If it happened to us, it could happen to anyone." He told fellow parents about the red flags he and his wife had missed, the questions they didn't ask, the things they wished they had known. "Our sole wish now is that no family has to go through what we're going through," they shared at her memorial service, "And that Aria's death has as much meaning as her life."

To our surprise, and unlike all the other suicide losses in Poplar Grove, Aria's death was not, to our knowledge, followed by other suicide deaths or even suicide attempts. Youth were distraught, to be sure, but none of our local mental health worker interlocutors shared information about a spike in suicide attempts among local youth after Aria's death—numbers (not names) they generally kept us fully updated about, given our roles as researchers in the community. So while we cannot be 100% certain that Aria's death was less socially contagious than others in the community, our data make it appear that way.

6.6.2 Talk Openly About the Pain of Grieving

Much of our time in Poplar Grove, along with other research, showed that exposure to suicide can increase youth's vulnerability to suicide through a force often called social contagion.[9,10] Exposure to suicide can change the meanings and motives youth ascribe to suicide in ways that may even shape youth's own behavioral repertoires, particularly when youth tightly identify with other youth's motives for suicide.[18] We expected to find that. And we heard that in Becca and Madison's testimonies.

What surprised us was how witnessing grief could lead to a kind of "social inoculation" for some youth in the very same community.[19] As with our cultural rebels, who in Chapter 2 demonstrated their ability to reject at least some of the town's narrow cultural expectations, we met youth like Chloe, Jack, and Shara, whose exposure to suicide seemed to offer them protection against suicidality. Social contagion pathways are more widely acknowledged and statistically significant,[9,10] but social inoculation arose as a hopeful counterweight, diminishing some youths' normative capacity for suicide after exposure.

And what was key to social inoculation? We found that it was witnessing *other people's* grief. Chloe's story helps us explain.

"After Kennedy did *that*, I would *never do that*," Chloe declared in our interview. She continued, forcefully:

I wouldn't do it to my mother. I wouldn't do it to my friends . . . Kennedy woke me up a little bit. . . . I might not have really grasped the importance and the beauty of the life that I had and have now, had I not recognized how quick and how ugly it can be when you lose someone. Especially [when you lose someone] in a selfish way. And I don't want to put that on anyone.

When we met her, in her early adulthood, Chloe was a successful businesswoman and proud homeowner living in nearby Binghamton. We couldn't help but assume she was one of those ideal-typical Poplar Grove youth, defined by the pursuit—and achievement—of personal and professional success. Through our interview, we learned that was true—but only to an extent. She *was* friends with everyone in high school, fluidly bouncing between social groups. She *was* gregarious and smart. But her adolescence was challenging. Chloe grew up in a single-parent home, where financial security and other markers of stability weren't quite "a thing."

Chloe and Kennedy were best friends in middle school, but Chloe's mental health took a nose dive much earlier than Kennedy's. By sixth grade, Chloe was hospitalized with an eating disorder. It wouldn't be the last time. In her words, her teenage years were angsty, and she had "a lot of issues going on." Suicide seemed obvious, like a universal aspect of the adolescent experience. "I can honestly say I think everyone, in their life, has contemplated suicide," she shared. But what had been idle, angsty thoughts changed dramatically when Chloe lost Kennedy to suicide.

This is where one might expect to read about Chloe struggling with her own suicidal thoughts, perhaps even attempting suicide. Instead, Kennedy's suicide seemed selfish to her—like Luke, she saw the terrible pain her friend's action caused for everyone left behind. It was also a powerful wakeup call about the precious nature of life. "I would never do that," Chloe declared with a sort of moral certainty. She felt Kennedy had been careless with the hearts and minds of those she loved, including Chloe's own mom, who grieved terribly for the girl she'd known since her early childhood. In a way, her best friend's death gave Chloe a weird opportunity to witness how her own death would impact her mother.

Kennedy's death "was really hard on my mom," Chloe began. In fits and starts, she continued, "I mean, like I said, she watched us grow up, together, so seeing someone grow up, and then losing them is—I mean, that was hard on her." Plus, Chloe's mom had weathered her own daughter's "rough adolescence" in which Kennedy had played such a helpful part, "the person that I was there with through the entire time . . ." For two and a half years, she said, her mom "thought that I was going to kill myself, or die from an eating disorder. . . . And, I made it through that storm . . . I mean, just barely. But, I did."

Kennedy, however, didn't. "And, I think that seeing Kennedy die just really—" Chloe paused, thinking of her mother's pain, then said, "She was preparing herself, I think, for if I ever did anything like that." Years later, the young woman and her mom still struggled with the loss. "We have a picture of Kennedy in our living room. . . . It's tucked away, but, every once in a [while] now, you happen to see it and it's like, 'Oh, hey Kennedy.' Like, she's still with us."

Jack was also Kennedy's friend, and he, too, became more reflective about suicide in the wake of her death. Suicide is "something I could never do," Jack explained, "because you just see the results; which is really the worst part. . . . There is . . . all this havoc it causes. . . . I mean, [Kennedy's parents] will never get over it."

Importantly, inoculation wasn't uniquely tied to experiencing personal grief. Regardless of their beliefs about suicide as selfish, an option, imaginable, understandable, or unacceptable, those who lost someone to suicide grieved. Some of those who experienced inoculation could deeply empathize with those who died; many felt a lot of anger, too. But what was unique to the youth we met who experienced inoculation was that they witnessed the grief of others. Usually, this was the grief of the parents of the child who died, or in Chloe's case, her own mother.

The power of witnessing other people's grief was such that some inoculated youth had not, in fact, lost a personally close contact to suicide.[19] Shara, for example, lost a number of schoolmates this way, but felt somewhat disconnected from their deaths. "One of the girls I went to high school with [Lauren], who I was an acquaintance with and hung out a few times, she committed suicide," Shara recounted. Then Shara and her family joined an Out of Darkness Walk, like the one we wrote about in the opening to this chapter. Shara joined the group walking in honor of Lauren, and there she met Lauren's mother.

"Lauren's mother was the sponsor for the group we were in," Shara explained, "and I just, when I met her . . . I kind of, like, realized the amount of just guilt and stress and emotions, and the toll that it takes on a family" when someone dies by suicide. Sandra, Lauren's mother, is warm and caring, a woman who wears her heart on her sleeve, and community suicide prevention events frequently bring tears to her eyes. She's quick to let kids see her pain—the devastation of losing a child to suicide. It's easy, in her presence, to move from wondering "What was so painful that Lauren had to end her life?" to "How could anyone do this to Sandra?"

Meeting Sandra, Shara confessed, "helped me to talk" about Shara's own mental health, and specifically her struggles with depression. "At least, like, I can talk to her about it. I can talk to someone about it who's dealt with it." By "it," she means the whole package of mental health problems, suicide, and the aftermath of suicide. Shara specified that she *wanted* to be reminded of what it would cost the people she loved if she, too, died by suicide. Like Jack and Chloe, she came to a similar understanding of suicide, but in a more vicarious way, through her involvement in suicide prevention efforts and interactions with those directly impacted by the deaths in her community. "*That's* what happens?" Shara exclaimed, as if reacting to Sandra's grief for the first time. "[I]t's like, 'Whoa, I don't want to do that.'"

This pattern of social inoculation that we found in Poplar Grove among some youth who witnessed the intense grieving of (generally) the parents of the youth who died can help us think through ways that memorialization can be safer. Being open about how terrible it hurts to lose your child to suicide may help other children be a little less likely to consider suicide as a means to escape unbearable psychological pain. Particularly when combined with open conversations about mental health, help-seeking, and suicide, as Shara experienced through the AFSP Out of Darkness Walk, this pathway may be our best hope to honor the memory of loved ones who died by suicide without triggering suicide contagion or amplifying the despair, alienation, and passivity in the face of psychological pain.

6.7 CONCLUSION

It is truly human, after the loss of a member of our community, to want to mourn them, to remember the person for all the good they embodied. It is cathartic and essential to being able to move on individually and reconstitute the collective without that member's corporeal presence. Yet it is also imperative, especially when the loss is a youth suicide, to mourn them safely, keeping in mind that this type of death is confusing and a cause of complicated grieving. It is challenging to not memorialize or glamorize their best virtues and qualities, but we found this central to a community's ability to effectively engage in postvention.

Tamping down on glorifying the decedent's life—on celebrating them—can feel unnatural, as can emphasizing honest, open conversations about suicide that shift attention from the person who is gone to the pain their suicide causes for those left behind. Certainly, in Poplar Grove, an embrace of this lesson was elusive. But Aria's death and her parents' response—along with the surprising absence of a suicide cluster's emergence in this case—demonstrates the promise of making the difficult but necessary shift and to reimagining what collective, safe mourning looks and feels like. To have a safer, more preventive memorial for a youth who has died by suicide, we encourage families and communities to talk openly about suicide, and about the visceral grief that accompanies suicide.

REFERENCES

1. Durkheim E. *The Elementary Forms of Religious Life*. New York: Free Press; 1912 [1995].
2. Turner V. *The Ritual Process: Structure and Anti-Structure*. Ithaca, NY: Cornell University Press; 1969.
3. Halbwachs M. *On Collective Memory*. Chicago: University of Chicago; 1992.
4. Olick JK, Robbins J. Social Memory Studies: From "Collective Memory" to the Historical Sociology of Mnemonic Practices. *Annual Review of Sociology*. 1998;24:105–140.
5. Diefendorf S, Van Norden S, Abrutyn S, Mueller AS. Understanding Suicide Bereavement, Contagion, and the Importance of Thoughtful Postvention in Schools. In: Ackerman JP, Horowitz LM, eds. *Youth Suicide Prevention and Intervention*. New York: Springer; 2022:51–60.
6. American Foundation for Suicide Prevention. *After a Suicide: A Toolkit for Schools*, 2nd ed. Waltham, MA: Education Development Center; 2018. Retrieved 6/24/22. https://afsp.org/after-a-suicide-a-toolkit-for-schools.
7. Hatfield E, Cacioppo JT, Rapson RL. *Emotional Contagion*. New York: Cambridge University Press; 1994.
8. Hatfield E, Rapson RL, Le YL. Emotional Contagion and Empathy. In: Decety J, Ickes W, eds. *The Social Neuroscience of Empathy*. Boston: MIT Press; 2009:19–30.
9. Abrutyn S, Mueller AS. Are Suicidal Behaviors Contagious? Using Longitudinal Data to Examine Suicide Suggestion. *American Sociological Review*. 2014;79(2):211–227.
10. Mueller AS, Abrutyn S. Suicidal Disclosures Among Friends: Using Social Network Data to Understand Suicide Contagion. *Journal of Health and Social Behavior*. 2015;56(1):131–148.
11. Klonsky ED, May A. Rethinking Impulsivity in Suicide. *Suicide and Life-Threatening Behavior*. 2010;40(6):612–619.
12. Klonsky ED, May AM. The Three-Step Theory (3ST): A New Theory of Suicide Rooted in the "Ideation-to-Action" Framework. *International Journal of Cognitive Therapy*. 2015;8(2):114–129.

13. Millner AJ, Robinaugh DJ, Nock MK. Advancing the Understanding of Suicide: The Need for Formal Theory and Rigorous Descriptive Research. *Trends in Cognitive Sciences*. 2020;24(9):704–716.

14. Auerbach RP, Stewart JG, Johnson SL. Impulsivity and Suicidality in Adolescent Inpatients. *Journal of Abnormal Child Psychology*. 2017;45:91–103.

15. Phillips JA, Luth EA. Beliefs About Suicide Acceptability in the United States: How Do They Affect Suicide Mortality? *The Journals of Gerontology: Series B*. 2020;75(2):414–425.

16. Renberg ES, Hjelmeland H, Koposov R. Building Models for the Relationship Between Attitudes Toward Suicide and Suicidal Behavior: Based on Data from General Population Surveys in Sweden, Norway, and Russia. *Suicide and Life-Threatening Behavior*. 2008;38(6):661–675.

17. Glenn CR, Millner AJ, Esposito EC, Porter AC, Nock MK. Implicit Identification with Death Predicts Suicidal Thoughts and Behaviors in Adolescents. *Journal of Clinical Child & Adolescent Psychology*. 2019;48(2):263–272.

18. Abrutyn S, Mueller AS, Osborne M. Rekeying Cultural Scripts for Youth Suicide: How Social Networks Facilitate Suicide Diffusion and Suicide Clusters Following Exposure to Suicide. *Society and Mental Health*. 2019;10(2):112–135. doi: 10.1177/2156869319834063.

19. Miklin S, Mueller AS, Abrutyn S, Ordoñez K. Suicide Exposure, Suicide Risk, and the Importance of Meaning Making. *Social Science and Medicine*. 2019;233:21–27.

7

ADDRESSING THE SOCIAL
ROOTS OF SUICIDE

We knew from the start we weren't asking a simple question: How is it possible that a vibrant, deeply connected, and caring community, filled with successful people and abundant resources, also suffers from an enduring youth suicide problem? We looked to the wisdom of youth, parents, mental health professionals, school staff, and other community members who, together, painted a picture of life and death in Poplar Grove. The overarching answer is that youth suicide is incredibly complex, but undeniably has social roots. That is, the social environment that kids inhabit in their everyday lives can exacerbate their risk of suicide, cause them psychological pain, and limit their ability to identify solutions other than suicide. If we fail to recognize or intervene in these social roots, our efforts at suicide prevention will likely be unsuccessful.

Accounting for the social environment in understanding youth suicide adds complexity to an already complex problem. But by sharpening our focus on the social worlds that youth inhabit, we can identify new opportunities for effective suicide prevention. This focus is consistent with long-standing public health approaches to prevention that seek to improve everyone's well-being rather than just the folks who need it most. For example, it encourages us to think about how to build social environments for youth that meet their psycho-social-developmental needs and enable them to thrive, regardless of what pressures, or stresses, or diagnosable mental illnesses they face. Let's build a strong foundation for childhood and adolescence so that when difficult times come—as they always have and always will—kids have the social and emotional resources to weather the storm.

There is rarely a single reason someone ends their life, or one thing we could have done to prevent their suicide. We join other scholars to advocate for a multifaceted, "upstream" approach to suicide prevention.[1] The analogy holds that, with a river flowing swiftly toward a dangerous waterfall, it is more effective to keep kids from falling into the river than trying to snatch them out at the very last moment, right before the waterfall (assuming we can even know when the very last moment is). Upstream approaches to suicide prevention encourage us to both identify youth in crisis and ensure they receive appropriate, life-affirming care *and* seek ways to help all kids.

In our years of investigation, speaking with communities, and careful study of youth and their social environments in and beyond Poplar Grove, we have learned many lessons. Not all towns are Poplar Grove, but what we learned there offers crucial insights that any community can use to better understand and address their local challenges with youth suicide. These insights can also point us toward new and effective intervention strategies for suicide that can work in Poplar Grove and inform suicide prevention in other places, too. In this closing chapter, we focus on the hopeful outcomes of a long and sometimes sad research journey, and we spend these last pages extracting tangible social and scientific lessons and offering concrete, evidence-informed steps for parents, schools, communities, and scientists to reduce kids' vulnerability to suicide.

7.1 LESSONS LEARNED

7.1.1 Lesson 1: Social Environments Shape Youth's Psychological Pain and Vulnerability to Suicide

While it is not news that the social environment matters to suicide, in this book, we elaborate our understanding of how the social worlds that kids and families inhabit matter to suicide risk and prevention. What we saw in Poplar Grove was that an ostensibly ideal social environment—a well-resourced town full of highly involved parents, excellent academic and athletic programs, substantial resources, and strong shared ideals about cultivating kids to their fullest potential—could, in fact, be a tinderbox. If a single suicide is a match, a seemingly idyllic town may be ready to go up in the flames of a suicide cluster—because of its social environment.

In Poplar Grove, several elements contributed to its vulnerability to recurring youth suicide clusters. The first was surprising. The high degree of social connectedness we found in Poplar Grove ultimately created problems for youth's psychological well-being. Everyone knew everyone, and everyone was expected to be a good neighbor, to keep a collective watch over the kids, to be ready to help each other with problems large and small. Kids shared this understanding of their community. Any adult was a resource that could be relied upon, at least for most things. These dense networks helped maintain a strong sense of pride in being from Poplar Grove. Many kids wanted to grow up and raise their own families in this ideal place, and many adults raising their families there had grown up in Poplar Grove themselves. While this sounds amazing—and in many ways it is—there are downsides to growing up in this tight-knit community.

The close, dense network ties encouraged judgmental gossip, a form of soft social control familiar to us all. Private, personal, sensitive information about kids and their families easily slipped into the public domain through these gossip networks. People knew who got the best scholarship into college, who was going to play Division I sports after high school, and who was struggling, who had been hospitalized for their mental health, or who was taking antidepressants. This gossip was particularly painful because Poplar Grovians had a clear understanding of what an ideal family looked like and what being an ideal Poplar Grove kid entailed. And it didn't include suicidal thoughts or mental health struggles. Kids felt pressure to be the perfect Poplar Grove kid. And that mostly meant being academically and athletically excellent, destined for a top-notch college—preferably on a merit scholarship—and a prestigious career. And the thing is, this goal felt tangible because so many Poplar Grove families were living out this esteemed life trajectory.

But these pressures to live up to community ideals—to achieve greatness—were not just individual family projects. It meant something to be from Poplar Grove as opposed to one of the other similarly nice, but just not quite as elite, communities in the county. Poplar Grove is described as one of the most desirable communities with the highest ranked public schools in not only Poplar Grove's county, but also the entire state. Community members were invested in this reputation. Families felt the pressure—make sure your kids help maintain the school's rank. The school felt the pressure—maintain your reputation for academic and athletic excellence. It is no wonder that kids also felt the pressure. Literally every single kid we talked to knew the mold of academic and preferably also athletic, or at least extracurricular, excellence they were supposed to fit.

In sum, pressure was great, expectations were narrow and clearly defined, and privacy was scarce. Kids and families knew if someone failed to meet expectations, it would be publicly known and talked about. And that was a terrifying reality for many. Because people *love* being from Poplar Grove. They love their community and take great pride in how they care for each other, pull toward common goals, and support each other through thick and thin—all the positive sides of life in the Grove. What was not obvious to locals is that this combination of high expectations and strong connectedness generated a silent threat for kids: if they failed, they would not belong to their cherished community and could be cast out. This threat of nonbelonging was painful for a lot of kids, and only a few kids—the ones we called our cultural rebels—managed to even somewhat reject the intense pressure to conform and compete, to achieve being a "good Poplar Grove kid."

We saw the consequences of these tight networks and perfection imperatives for kids, both in those who attempted or died by suicide and in those who were left confused when the seemingly "perfect" kid to whom they compared themselves died by suicide. Our interviews found the so-cial environment kids navigated daily was saturated with a fear of failure, individualized to the point of personal pathology, and private shame at-tached to the ways they perceived they were failing or deficient, unde-serving of community membership. In other words, the shadowy side of the culture of excellence was a culture of shame and embarrassment at any possible imperfection. While youth who died by suicide often had other things going on in their lives—including sometimes diagnosable mental illnesses—we found evidence that their psychological pain, or their shame at their failures (e.g., problems at college), or their contact with law en-forcement was exacerbated by their sense of who they should be and their failure to measure up to that ideal.

Ultimately, Poplar Grove reveals much about how the social environ-ment can condition youth's psychological pain. This general lesson can be broken down into two sublessons. The first is that connectivity can be won-derful and protective, *or* it can feel overwhelming, stifling, suffocating, and precarious. Highly connected groups can demand too much from their members, such that the duties and obligations of membership become un-bearable expectations.[2] They do this by fostering internal, informal con-trol in the form of peer or neighborly monitoring. A knowing look, the threat of gossip—these are easy and cheap ways to enforce social rules. They also heighten the perceived consequences of nonconformity; the threat of sanctions is exceptionally painful when the community provides a wealth of positive effects, like belongingness, attention, affection, and well-defined acceptable roles, identities, and behaviors.[3,4] Together, these aspects lead individuals to self-monitor their moral alignment, which we all know is enormously hard on our emotional and psychological health and wellness.[5]

This leads to the second sublesson. Narrow cultural beliefs are painful for those who do not fit in.[6,7] Poplar Grove is not alone in this down-side to their wonderful sense of community. There are many examples of narrow cultural beliefs increasing the vulnerability of some to suicidal ideation and action. Narrow beliefs about acceptable forms of masculinity, for example, are associated with greater risk of suicidality among men who see themselves as failing to perform the "right" kind of manhood.[8,9] Similarly, in China, there has been an epidemic of suicide among rural married women, and researchers have shown that this epidemic is tied to rigid community rules about what a dutiful wife feels, thinks, and does, combined with few options for how wives can remedy or escape family situations that feel unfair or unjust.[10,11] And in the United States, the guiding ideals of heterosexuality and binary gender norms—and their requirement for belonging in some communities, religions, and families— have led to disproportionately high rates of suicidal ideation, attempts, and likely, deaths among the lesbian, gay, bisexual, transgender, and queer (LGBTQ+) population.[12–15]

These examples also highlight one way that insights from our research in Poplar Grove on the social roots of suicide can transfer to other communities, even if they look very different from Poplar Grove. While the content of the narrow cultural beliefs or directives may vary, wherever we find narrow cultural ideals we find people who struggle to fit the mold, who feel they do not belong. And they are likely suffering. Limited "appropriate" choices amplify distress, psychological pain, and thus, vulnerability to suicide, particularly when combined with gossip about who doesn't fit in or meet community expectations. Identifying and addressing the narrow cultural beliefs and discouraging the gossip and social comparisons that together hinder belonging will help in any community's project to improve suicide prevention.

For suicide prevention, *Lesson 1* suggests a set of related, affirmative efforts to ensure youth encounter cultures of belonging and acceptance in their schools, families, faith communities, and neighborhoods. First, actively cultivating a culture of belonging for all—regardless of their social identities, demographic characteristics, talents, or interests—is a powerful antidote to narrow cultural beliefs. One way that schools and communities can do this is to make sure that public, formal celebrations of youth feature diverse metrics of success. Rather than publishing the quarterly honor roll, as Poplar Grove High School (PGHS) does, why not develop other recognitions—like the kindest student? Research has shown that adults have a lot of power to confer visibility and prominence on youth—through who is featured at pep rallies, graduations, in newsletters, and on websites—that matter to the adolescent members of school communities. This is why it's not surprising that Poplar Grove's kids value Advanced Placement courses as much as the adults in their community.[16] We can use these tools and rewards to shift youth cultures to acknowledge healthier, broader definitions of "success."

Second, states can also support building cultures of belonging by reinforcing federal laws with state laws. All kids have a fundamental right to feel welcomed, supported, and accepted at school. While federal law prevents discrimination or harassment on the basis of a variety of protected classes—including those based on race/ethnicity, religion, immigrant status, and gender—some states have taken this a step further. Colorado, Illinois, and California, to name just a few, have additionally elaborated who is protected and in what instances at school, helping to ensure that all kids, including gender and sexual minorities, have an equal opportunity to participate and thrive at school without harrassment (see www.lgbtmap.org). Legislation to protect the well-being of all kids, regardless of their social identities, gives schools and communities the fundamental tools needed to build and enforce inclusive policies.[17]

Third, there are existing educational interventions—like Challenge Success (www.challengesuccess.org)—that target narrow beliefs around academic excellence and address academic pressure.[18] In places like Poplar Grove, Challenge Success and other interventions like it, while not originally conceived of as suicide prevention interventions, may help improve youth mental health and prevent suicide. Incidentally, Challenge Success also addresses concerns about connectivity and gossip by offering a framework to encourage privacy and discourage social comparisons on academic metrics. While we have no ties to Challenge Success (or any other interventions we mention in this chapter), what we like about Challenge Success is that it is also a community intervention—students, schools, and parents all have roles to play in building a community with more diverse views of success and less academic pressure.

7.1.2 Lesson 2: Mental Health Stigma Thwarts Help-Seeking and Undermines Suicide Prevention

While the social connectedness and narrow beliefs played a major role in youth suicide in Poplar Grove, another toxic cousin worked in tandem to suppress help-seeking among kids and their families: mental health stigma. Having mental health struggles or a mental illness was stigmatized in Poplar Grove as antithetical to being that ideal kid or that ideal family. "Good" kids and "good" families just didn't have depression, anxiety, or experience psychological pain. To seek help for one of these problems was seen as an admission of imperfection, which flagrantly violated the directive to achieve—and achieve perfectly. Grafted onto the local culture of excellence, mental health stigma, so rampant in the United States, meant that kids worked to hide their struggles, parents worked to ignore the signs of those struggles, and families suppressed information about their problems. This was amplified by the fact that help-seeking was believed to be an incitement to gossip and social sanctioning. If you went to therapy or took an antidepressant, the whole world would know. And when families had children that absolutely needed mental health help, they felt like they had to keep the problem quiet. The air of silence that hung around many families with kids in therapy or inpatient hospitalization isolated those families. The caring, supportive community that defined life in Poplar Grove was suddenly gone, often when families needed it most, because of this silence. While some of this was self-imposed by those families, they heard the gossip, they knew what people said, so it wasn't irrational—just unfortunate.

It is not surprising, then, that when kids experienced increasing psychological pain or suicidal despair, they did not see asking for help as a real option. Those marvelous social networks, so rich in care and concern and love for every other problem under the sun, were not considered as sources of support when the problem that needed to be discussed was mental health related. "The thought [of telling my friends about my mental health issues] never crossed my mind," Felicity, a young adult who survived a serious suicide attempt during her high school years, told us.

And yet Felicity is absolutely sure that her friends would have been there for her, if she had only asked. Indeed, after almost losing her life, her friends swarmed her with love and kindness and still remain her closest confidants today, years later.

Felicity's story is emblematic of youth who attempted or died by suicide in Poplar Grove —getting help just wasn't an option. If we are thinking about suicide prevention, this is just as problematic as having a social environment that exacerbates youth's psychological pain and risk of sui- cide. Problems happen. Things cause us pain. Some of us develop mental illnesses. It's just a part of life. We cannot be happy-go-lucky 100% of the time. But when a community stigmatizes these experiences of psycho- logical pain or mental illness as ruining an entire person's worth—what sociologist Erving Goffman called spoiling their identity[19]—it can make it incredibly difficult to recognize that the psychological pain deserves life-affirming healthcare and support. It can also make it difficult to rec- ognize that one's life isn't over when mental illness descends. And that treatment, management, and even recovery are possible outcomes when feeling the onset of major depression or other illnesses. Growing up in a context where mental health stigma abounds thwarts help-seeking, which in turn raises youth's risk of suicide.

If we want to prevent suicide effectively, we cannot neglect mental health stigma. We can build the most robust mental health safety nets, but no kids or families will use them unless we make it safe and comfort- able to seek help. Luckily, there are many existing interventions that help schools and their communities end mental health stigma. Two evidence- based examples in the United States are Bring Change to Mind[20] (www. bringchange2mind.org) and Sources of Strength (https://sourcesofstren gth.org).[1]

One family in Poplar Grove also powerfully role-modeled another way to move the dial on mental health stigma: talk openly about mental health challenges. Two parents of a girl who died by suicide—Josie and Will Stephens—were very open about their daughter Aria's mental health struggles, at her memorial service and beyond. They talked passion- ately and honestly about their own diagnosed mental illnesses and Aria's probable diagnosis. They talked about what it is like to live with mental illness, how treatment can help, and how mental illnesses are just like any other health problem. Mental illness, along with any mental health struggle, deserves respect, care, and treatment, not shame and silence. For many, Josie and Will's open and honest discussions created space for conversations that ended silences. As a result, close friends admitted that their own children were struggling with mental health. Finally, that wonderful community safety net was freed to wrap support around those families and kids. They were shown love out in the open instead feeling shame in the dark. This is a powerful antidote to mental health stigma. And all it takes is for each of us to share our stories. Because many of us have faced challenges with our mental health, if more of us role-model how we cope, how we seek help, then hopefully more of us will feel that healing is possible and that suicide is not our only option.

7.1.3 Lesson 3: Authentically Caring School-Based Postvention Is Critical

The cultural values of achievement and excellence in Poplar Grove, along with the mental health stigma and the shared concern over the community's reputation, also harmed efforts to help youth and the community heal after suicide losses. Losing someone to suicide is a terribly painful experience, perhaps particularly for youth who may be experiencing death for the first time. And when a youth is exposed to either the suicide attempt or suicide death of a friend, they are, on average, at increased risk of developing suicidal thoughts and attempting suicide.[21] Exposure to suicide carries risk, but it is a risk that can be ameliorated through thoughtful "postvention."

Because schools are the center of adolescents' social lives, schools are broadly considered one of the most important places for youth suicide prevention and for compassionate, caring suicide postvention.[22,23] In PGHS's postvention approaches, we saw repeated problems that generated a divide between youth and school staff and a sense among kids that they and their peers didn't really matter. Over time, as suicide postvention guidelines improved, PGHS and its school district adopted some recommendations (namely, recommendations from *After a Suicide, A Toolkit for Schools*[22]), but PGHS's postvention responses were still primarily guided by fear—generally, fear that their actions might trigger another suicide cluster, for which they would be blamed. This fear seemed to paralyze the school and make inaction seem like a safer choice than the actions suggested by guidebooks.[24] Rather than focusing on promoting healing, acknowledging what had happened, and providing information about suicide, mental health, and help-seeking, the school focused on moving on as quickly as possible. Suicide was not talked about after suicide losses happened, or even at other times during the school year. Seats were not consistently or respectfully rearranged in classrooms to fill voids left behind by missing classmates. Crisis counselors were called in and available, but the strategies to ensure kids in need found their way to mental health supports were not dependable. Many kids slipped through the cracks. And when kids did find their way to crisis counselors, their needs were not always prioritized, and follow-up was not the best even when kids really needed it.

Lesson 3 has implications for improving school's postvention strategies. For school-based postvention, the first step is for schools and their school districts to plan ahead and be prepared to execute an evidence-informed suicide postvention strategy. The resource *After a Suicide*[22] provides important guidance on how to do this, but we have a few added suggestions. First, some of the guidelines in *After a Suicide* are vague, particularly in the real-world context of a postvention response. This means that schools always have to make tough day-of decisions, often under significant time pressure, no matter how well prepared they are. To help make those decisions, we recommend that the school's orienting principle during postvention be to take care of kids' mental health in an authentic and supportive manner. Making sure every decision is filtered through this principle, we believe, will go a long way toward ensuring that the school's response is as safe and helpful as possible. It is categorically unacceptable for suicide postvention to be "more awkward" (as Poplar Grove's district cautioned it would be) than other crisis responses. In Poplar Grove, the acceptance of awkwardness in postvention resulted from their fear that talking openly and honestly about suicide would trigger suicide clusters. But the opposite was likely true. Awkwardness and silence are at odds with compassionate and authentic caring. They are at odds with what kids need to feel safe and heal in these moments of vulnerability. Suicide postvention has to be as warm and caring and supportive as any response to a death that impacts the school community. Given the complexities of suicide prevention and postvention, the best we can do is distill things down to a guiding principle and use that when in doubt.

Second, when a suicide death is the latest in a long line of suicides, or when suicide clusters are recurring in a school or a community, it is very necessary for the school district to acknowledge what is happening and take active steps to improve suicide pre- and postvention. Reputations will not be saved by trying to ignore the reality of what's happening. Risks will increase with silence. In addition to the postvention resources already mentioned, the American Foundation for Suicide Prevention (AFSP) has an entire webpage devoted to programs that schools can use to incorporate suicide prevention into schooling.[25] The Suicide Prevention Resource Center also hosts a registry of evidence-based programs that can be used with youth of different ages and in schools.[26] We also refer regularly to the book *Suicide in Schools* when we are guiding schools on suicide prevention or postvention.[24]

Third, one of the best ways to prevent suicide is to talk about suicide, and schools are one of the most important places where we can educate students about suicide, including the warning signs for suicide, how to talk to peers or an adult about suicidal thoughts, and how to seek help for oneself or a friend. The silence around suicide in Poplar Grove was awful for kids. It created its own fear and anxiety, above and beyond the repeated suicide losses. And while the community of Poplar Grove occasionally hosted suicide gatekeeper trainings, kids rarely showed up. If we think this information is important and life-saving—which we certainly do—then it needs to become part of kids' curriculum in their schools. There are plenty of options for incorporating curriculum about suicide into schooling, and while time is always scarce during the school day, we feel investing in kids' mental health is worth it.

Fourth, sometimes students may want to memorialize their friend who died by suicide at school in ways that may not be in line with best practices. We saw this in Poplar Grove. When this happens, whenever possible, school staff should talk with students and families about the honest reasons why a request for memorialization must be denied rather than just shutting kids down without explanation. Again, holding close to that orienting principle of helping kids heal and demonstrating authentic caring for kids, as these conversations are held, will help tremendously. We find that explaining concerns to students and families goes a long way toward building understanding, and that students *can* understand. Students also do not want to live through the experience of a suicide cluster. They care deeply about protecting their friends. It may also help if school staff redirect students' and parents' efforts to a safer but still meaningful way to memorialize the student who died; something we pick up next in *Lesson 4*. We also want to acknowledge that even if schools follow all recommendations, including our suggested guiding principle, some parents and some students will likely still be unhappy or even blame the school. We will return to this issue in *Lesson 6*.

7.1.4 Lesson 4: Safer Memorialization Happens When Suicide Is Not Romanticized and Instead Is Discussed Openly

Memorial services for youth who died by suicide in Poplar Grove generally were disconcerting for youth. Messages at these services rarely mentioned suicide or even mental health—the things kids told us they most cared about. Unlike during the school's postvention response, this was not done out of fear of instigating a suicide cluster; rather, it was a consequence of the community's concern about reputation. The mental health stigma and local cultural ideals about good families and good children likely made it difficult to talk openly about suicide in the aftermath of a suicide loss, since suicide was interpreted as a mark of shame or imperfection on the child and their family's reputation. This culture of silence and mental health stigma meant that the focus at memorials was generally on celebrating the short but magnificent life of the youth who died. A surprising number of the youth who died by suicide were popular, seemingly perfect kids—kids who had it all. So at these events, which were attended by hundreds if not thousands of youth, the silence surrounding the cause of death meant that what kids repeatedly saw was that a perfect kid's life could just end one day, inexplicably by their own hand, and that the whole community would pour out to honor them. Youth explained to us that this sent an odd and confusing message; in this context, suicide seemed like a way to obtain the attention and love that kids sometimes feel is inaccessible in life due to the great expectations and high standards of Poplar Grove. It romanticized suicide as an option. It also reinforced mental health stigma and made it clear that suicide and mental health are things that shouldn't be talked about, even when it was incredibly, powerfully salient. And even when it was the very thing that brought them to the memorial service.

Kids noticed this disconnect. And it made them afraid. Who could be next? What if they just woke up one day and felt suicidal? These were real concerns kids in Poplar Grove shared with us. Rather than knowing how to talk about mental health and how to seek help when needed, kids felt collectively gaslit. This terrible thing kept happening, but no one would acknowledge it. Instead, adults seemed to celebrate it at memorial services through the incredible attendance and showers of attention on the youth who died by suicide. While in reality no adults were celebrating the repeating youth suicides, the point we are trying to convey is that, to vulnerable youth, it seemed as though they were. We aren't sure it's a good idea to change the number of people who show up at a memorial service to mourn a person who has passed away—memorial services are important for processing grief, and we would not want to deny that to anyone who felt impacted—but we can change what is said at the memorial service so that we do not leave kids with the collective sense that suicide is a way to gain prominence in a world where prominence feels so important and hard to come by. We can talk about suicide. We can talk about psychological pain.

Let us be very clear: research has repeatedly shown that talking about suicide does not cause suicide and likely protects against it.[27] Bringing suicide out of the silence is the safer choice. It's also the only choice—because kids will talk amongst themselves. They will not be silent. The only option for adults is whether we join in the conversation.

We saw one example in Poplar Grove of adults including discussions of mental health in memorial services. And the example was a powerful one. The Stephens, who lost their daughter Aria to suicide, as we mentioned earlier, were quite open about Aria's mental health struggles at her memorial service and beyond. They were also very open about their own grief and how devastated their family was by Aria's death by suicide. Watching the terrible pain of families mourning their child's suicide actually had a powerful—and surprising—effect on youth in Poplar Grove. One of the strongest patterns in our data, stronger even than the more well-known and feared social contagion effect, was what we call a social inoculation effect. When kids witnessed the grief of the family who lost their child to suicide, many reported emphatically that suicide was *not* an option for them, even kids who had previously had suicidal thoughts. Kids told us that by witnessing the family's grief, they developed a greater understanding of just what losing a child to suicide does to a family. They extrapolated from that what their own death by suicide would do to their own family, and realized they could never destroy their family like that. This pattern suggests memorials that talk about suicide, mental health, and help-seeking, and that do not hide the pain of losing a child to suicide specifically, may actually help kids understand suicide in a new way—a way that protects kids from suicide.

We acknowledge that it can be hard to dictate how suicide or mental health is talked about at memorial services, where grieving families guide the event. But if it is possible, we found in Poplar Grove that it was powerfully helpful. Since it won't always be possible, it is even more important to have these conversations in other moments and locations. That way, if kids attend a memorial service for someone who has died by suicide and mental health and suicide are not mentioned, or are mentioned in a harmful and stigmatizing way, kids have some basis for making sense of suicide that is broader than the messages they receive at the memorial service. This takes us back to *Lesson 3* on the importance of embedding suicide prevention curriculum in schools. We have to make sure that kids get the information they need about suicide and mental health.

Lesson 4 has implications for how we can construct safer mourning rituals and memorial services. First, and most notably, we believe safer memorialization is achieved by bringing suicide, or at least mental health and mental health help-seeking, into the conversation during mourning rituals. If nothing else, avoiding stigmatizing or shaming language during the memorial service is important. But addressing suicide more explicitly, if possible, can powerfully change the tone and the lessons kids take away from memorial services and vigils, especially when tied to the pain of the family left behind.

Second, because talking about suicide and mental health in accurate and nonstigmatizing ways is essential to safer memorialization, ensuring that informed, trained, caring people are present to offer evidence-informed guidance is critically important. Because faith communities are often in-volved in memorialization and mourning rituals, they must be prepared to respond to suicide losses in evidence-informed ways.[28] In Poplar Grove, the faith communities were aware of their importance and often appeared as up-to-date on best practices as possible. It just wasn't always enough to counteract the community's local culture. But the suicide research commu-nity could also do better. We have not been as attentive to the needs of faith communities during postvention as we have been to the needs of schools. The guidebook for faith leaders—*After a Suicide: Recommendations for Religious Services*[26]—has not been updated since 2004, despite advances in our understanding of healing after a suicide. There is also very little research devoted to understanding postvention and memorialization in faith communities.

Third, Out of Darkness Walks organized by local chapters of the AFSP may be an important way to safely honor loved one's memories without romanticizing suicide. Before we discuss why, we will acknowledge that we have a conflict of interest with AFSP, since they funded our research from 2019 to 2021 (including part of this study), and they raise funds for research and other activities through these Walks. Still, we are confident that our support of these Walks is rooted in our research and not our past research funding. In Poplar Grove, there is a great need to not forget the youth who have died by suicide and to acknowledge the pain of their passing. This need is evidenced in the number of teenagers who show up for the annual Out of Darkness Walk decked out in team t-shirts honoring their friend who died by suicide. Every youth we spoke with who attended or was involved in these events found it a helpful way to honor their loved one's memory.

One advantage of AFSP-sponsored Out of Darkness Walks is that trained suicide prevention experts from the local AFSP chapter are generally present to provide information about warning signs for suicide and how to get help. The Walks in Poplar Grove often start with talks about suicide loss, healing, and prevention. As a result, the memorialization— the t-shirts and wristbands that kids wear to embody their grief—goes hand in hand with an emphasis on and conversation about suicide prevention. The event itself also helps address mental health stigma by everyone showing up to bring attention to the very thing that usually receives so much silence—suicide. Perhaps hosting Out of Darkness Walks, which we have even seen high schools do (outside of Poplar Grove), is a meaningful and safer way to memorialize those we have lost and acknowledge the mental health challenges of being a kid in the 21st century, especially if local suicide prevention experts and crisis counselors are present.

Memorialization is important to healing, so we must hold spaces in our community to collectively acknowledge pain and loss. Our fears about suicide clusters should not cause us to avoid honoring the memory of someone who has died by suicide. But talking about suicide can be hard, and we, as a society rife with mental health and suicide stigma, often get it wrong. The more we prepare as communities, and the more we train community members to talk about suicide and mental health in open, honest, and nonstigmatizing ways, the better prepared we will be to create healing spaces where memory, grief, healing, and suicide prevention can coexist safely.

7.1.5 Lesson 5: Informed, Supported, and Empowered Youth Are Critical Suicide Prevention Leaders

Lessons 1 to 4, together, point to a need to include young people in community-level discussions about and approaches to suicide response. Youth are part of the social environment in which they are raised and in which their peers are dying. And they are part of the social fabric of kids supporting kids in the wake of suicides. They have firsthand experience that adults need to take seriously if they hope to disrupt a suicide problem. In short, kids are a key resource in suicide prevention.

The best strategies to prevent youth suicide must include a focus on empowering youth to build the cultures of mental wellness and belonging *they* feel they need.[23,29,30] Youth in Poplar Grove were quite clear about the sources of their psychological pain and what in their school and community needed changing. They tried to make their pain known to adults but were dismissed, likely due to those adults' preconceived notions about children, parenting, schooling, and the very fact that their town had a problem with youth suicide. This scenario was, honestly, at direct odds with the community's purported goals of preparing youth for the transition to successful adulthoods and raising future leaders. Kids were trying to lead, and they were brushed aside.

Youth are capable of so much more. Ageism is not only about discrimination against older individuals (as in job markets, where younger candidates are typically preferred), but also about documented prejudices regarding the agency and capabilities of children and youth. In one palpable example to the contrary, the youth survivors of a rampage shooting at Florida's Marjory Stoneman Douglas High School[31] spurred a national protest movement and changed the national conversation from a problem with mass shootings to a problem with gun violence. Youth are capable. Listening to youth and being respectful of their ability to educate adults on their lives is, at a broader level, important because their lives are radically different from our own at their age (just think of the rise of social media, the advance of climate change, and of course, the dramatic increase in rampage school shootings). When adults don't try to "get it" on kids' terms, youth lose trust in adults. And having trust in adults is one of the most powerful protective factors against youth suicide.[30] When youth trust adults, we can better prevent suicide. But we have to earn and maintain their trust.

Empowering youth goes beyond giving them a seat at the table. Their voices must be included in the design and implementation of suicide prevention, their ideas and perspectives must be taken as seriously as any other scientific data, and they must be able to take up leadership roles. Just like adults, they will require expert guidance to avoid exacerbating potentially harmful biases and assumptions in the solutions they innovate. But we are confident their innovations and insights will be worthwhile.

For suicide prevention, *Lesson 5* suggests communities consider youth front-line prevention experts, with direct knowledge and insights that no intervention strategy is complete without. Existing school-based intervention strategies provide frameworks for effectively engaging youth in suicide prevention and mental health promotion. Some we've mentioned before—like Bring Change to Mind[19] and Sources of Strength[1]—but there are others that can be found on the AFSP webpage and beyond.

7.1.6 Lesson 6: Schools and Infrastructure Are Important Targets for Scarce Public Funding

The fact that suicide prevention experts—including ourselves—endorse schools as fundamental to suicide prevention and mental health safety nets smacks directly into the fact that US schools typically experience intense resource scarcity.[32] This scarcity has, in many cases, risen to new heights since 2008, just as youth suicide rates have risen. While Poplar Grove's state does not have the most egregious decline in school funding over this period, their school funding has declined. At the same time, Poplar Grove's state has passed suicide prevention legislation that requires school staff members be trained regularly in suicide prevention. That sounds great. Public schools are wonderful places to start when it comes to kids' mental health, because they serve the whole community and, as we've learned, mental health and suicide are community-level issues. Kids spend the bulk of every weekday under the care of school staff, and a great portion of their evenings and weekends nested in the peer communities established by their grade levels and classes. Their parents have differing abilities to engage in communicating about mental health and suicide at home.

An intentional, well-resourced prevention strategy is, in fact, a perfect fit for school settings, but few schools have either. The official government fiscal policy note evaluating the new suicide prevention bill in Poplar Grove's state, for example, recognizes explicitly that the legislation imposes a mandate on schools that may increase local school system expenditures without providing any funding to do so. We are literally asking schools to do more with less when our children's lives are on the line. This sets up schools and school staff for terrible choices, for individuals taking on more than they can manage,[33] more than they are trained to do,[34] and more than school budgets can accommodate.

This scenario has implications for suicide prevention. Without proper funding, schools cannot increase the number of school counselors, psychologists, social workers, or other mental health support staff on campus, nor can they take advantage of evidence-based staff training programs, from the two-hour LivingWorks Start program to the PREPaRE program for school-based crisis response to the longer LivingWorks Applied Suicide Intervention Skills Training (ASIST) and beyond. Particularly if we as communities are going to get upset when schools do a less-than-perfect job at an incredibly difficult task, like suicide postvention—something we have seen far too often—it's important that we recognize our community's role in enabling schools to do this work well. They cannot do it without adequate resources. And we should not demand the world of school staff if we are also not going to make their lives livable by providing them the resources they need to support students in the 21st century.

Infrastructure funding, too, deserves more than a passing glance when it comes to suicide prevention. Means restriction is an important component of suicide prevention,[34] though we find that the public tends to misunderstand its purpose and downplay its effectiveness. Often, we have been told, "If someone wants to die, they're going to find a way." That may be true: research shows, for example, that some people whose access to guns is restricted will turn to alternative methods. But those alternative methods may be less lethal; thus, the person is less likely to die by suicide.

But this way of arguing against means restriction actually misses the point. The main goal of means restriction is not just to thwart one method of suicide; rather, it is to increase the time between the pain of a suicidal crisis and an action that may end a person's life. Suicidal crises do generally pass, so extending that time gap really matters. This is why medicine lockboxes and gun safes are effective: even if there is some way to break into them, they slow down suicidal actions. Sometimes time is all that is needed to avert suicide.

Public infrastructure matters as much as any gun lock mechanism: bridge barriers, for instance, are effective in stopping suicide at public landmarks.[36,37] In Poplar Grove, there is one particular bridge used by youth and adults to die by suicide. It has suicide prevention signage erected, yet it continues to contribute to tragedy. Community members are now working toward funding bridge barriers, a notoriously costly but effective form of public infrastructure for suicide prevention. We are cheering them on in their evidence-based efforts.

Lesson 6 suggests communities acknowledge the risk of youth (and adult) suicide and incorporate risk reduction into funding decisions regarding schools, community education, and public space. This is an era of dwindling public funding and overstretched budgets, but the answer cannot be allowing the public itself to dwindle. This is one instance in which money really can help. We additionally endorse legislation to mandate high-quality, evidence-based suicide prevention and means-restriction trainings for youth-involved adults (like school staff), but we encourage states to not make these laws unfunded mandates. Do not ask schools to do more with less. We also encourage families to use medicine and gun safes and for communities to make these life-saving resources available for free (or at as low a cost as feasible). Just as Poplar Grove's local library offered free COVID-19 tests to promote public health during a global pandemic, they could offer gun locks and medicine lockboxes with informative pamphlets on how and why to use them.

7.2 WHAT CAN YOU DO TODAY?

To turn the tide on youth suicide in Poplar Grove, and in the United States overall, is going to take major policy interventions, but it's also going to take each and every one of us deciding to get engaged. Most importantly, we all need to build competence in talking about suicide and mental health in effective and nonstigmatizing ways. This isn't easy. We all share a lot of understandable fears and cultural biases when it comes to these topics, but we have recommendations that can help along the way. We also urge you to not let the perfect be the enemy of the good. When you get hung up on when and what to say to whom and how, let empathy guide you. Active compassionate listening goes a long way.

7.2.1 Action 1: Speak Openly About Personal and Community Mental Health and Wellness

To help end mental health stigma and promote help-seeking, one of the most powerful things you can do is to speak out, including sharing your own story of mental illness or journey to mental wellness. The more we talk about valuing our own well-being, the more we normalize mental health struggles and mental health help-seeking, putting them on par with physical health problems, the better our suicide prevention efforts will be. Speaking openly can also help others recognize us as safe, trustworthy confidants for when they may need to talk to someone about their own mental health help. It's also okay to not wait for others to seek us out. Look for appropriate moments to inquire about others' health and well-being and offer your support. Sometimes just asking "hey, how are you doing truly?" and holding space for an honest answer can be powerful. Sharing our own mental health stories and starting mental health conversations are forms of vulnerability that build strength.

7.2.2 Action 2: Educate Yourself About Mental Health and Suicide Prevention

Many of the trainings mentioned in the *Lessons* of this chapter are good choices for educators and community members seeking a role in the prevention of youth suicide (e.g., LivingWorks ASIST training). Each will help you develop a vocabulary and templates for talking about suicide. If you have the time and resources, you won't regret participating in any of the modules recommended here or other suicide prevention trainings listed on AFSP's website.

Others can start their suicide prevention education with as little as 14 minutes—by listening to a short episode of the appropriately named science podcast *Short Wave* that covers the major steps in getting help for a loved one at risk of suicide.[38] It is full of factually correct information that dovetails with our own recommendations, and it is recent enough to reflect up-to-date best practices in the world of suicidology.

Additionally, Dr. Stacey Freedenthal, a clinician, professor, and suicide expert, has made a number of essays on suicide prevention freely available. These include our favorites "What NOT to Say" and "10 Things to Say" to a suicidal person, and they are accessible at speakingofsuicide.org. She also just published a book on what family, friends, and partners can say and do to support their loved one with suicidal thoughts.[39]

Talking about suicide directly and clearly saves lives, but we all need help learning how to talk about such a difficult and consequential topic. Other resources—like the trainings and readings we recommend—will help you spot subtle warning signs, such as changes in sleep patterns (see Chapter 3) that merit discussion. And as we noted earlier in the book, subtle signs may be the only ones we get that someone we care about is at risk for suicide.

7.2.3 Action 3: Cultivate a Destigmatizing, Empathic Approach to Talking About Suicide

Making sure that our own language doesn't inadvertently stigmatize mental health help-seeking or mental illness is important, and the guides presented in this chapter are helpful when it comes to evolving best practices. But again, though we know that words matter, empathy and active listening can bridge the gaps in our own knowledge. Cultivating empathy and just listening to people's stories goes a long way toward building a kinder, more caring world. We don't always have to understand everything about a person's illness or experiences to recognize their pain, express concern, and offer support. It may feel intrusive or nosey, but in fact, it is the opposite of gossipy grapevines and passive prying when you open up a conversation, no matter how messy, and offer your care.

7.3 CONCLUSION

When we began this work a decade ago, we had no idea where we would end up. At times, it is daunting and mentally taxing—surely this is the case for you, the reader, as well. Frequently, however, it is hopeful. We have been motivated by the urgent need to better understand and explain youth suicide so that communities, schools, families, and youth themselves have better information about and strategies through which to reduce the risk and pain of suicide. In the end, our wish is that our efforts have brought some comfort to any reader who is suffering, feeling alone or like a failure, as well as some invigoration to those social scientists who share our goals and some actionable preventive strategies to communities and community members affected by the collective trauma of suicide problems. Our words and deeds can save lives.

REFERENCES

1. Wyman PA, Brown CH, LoMurray M, et al. An Outcome Evaluation of the Sources of Strength Suicide Prevention Program Delivered by Adolescent Peer Leaders in High Schools. *American Journal of Public Health.* 2010;100(9):1653–1661.
2. Abrutyn S, Mueller AS. Towards a Cultural-Structural Theory of Suicide: Examining Excessive Regulation and its Discontents. *Sociological Theory.* 2018;36(1):48–66.
3. Swann Jr. WB, Jetten J, Gómez Á, Whitehouse H, Bastian B. When Group Membership Gets Personal: A Theory of Identity Fusion. *Psychological Review.* 2012;119(3):441–456.
4. Thoits PA. Multiple Identities and Psychological Well-Being: A Reformulation and Test of the Social Isolation Hypothesis. *American Sociological Review.* 1983;48(2):174–187.
5. Link BG, Phelan JC. Labeling and Stigma. In: Aneshenel CS, Phelan JC, Bierman A, eds. *The Handbook of the Sociology of Mental Health.* New York: Springer; 2013:525–541.
6. Abrutyn S. Toward a Sociological Theory of Social Pain. *Journal for the Theory of Social Behaviour.* 2023;53(3):351–371. doi: 10.1111/jtsb.12371.
7. Crosnoe R. *Fitting In, Standing Out: Navigating the Social Challenges of High School to Get an Education.* Cambridge, UK: Cambridge University Press; 2011.
8. Adinkrah M. Better Dead than Dishonored: Masculinity and Male Suicidal Behavior in Contemporary Ghana. *Social Science and Medicine.* 2012;74:474–481.
9. Cleary A. *The Gendered Landscape of Suicide: Masculinities, Emotions, and Culture.* London: Palgrave; 2019.
10. Fei W. *Suicide and Justice: A Chinese Perspective.* London: Routledge; 2010.
11. Manning J. *Suicide: The Social Causes of Self-Destruction.* Charlottesville, VA: University of Virginia Press; 2020.
12. Puckett JA, Woodward EN, Mereish EH, Pantalone DW. Parental Rejection Following Sexual Orientation Disclosure: Impact on Internalized Homophobia, Social Support, and Mental Health. *LGBT Health.* 2015;2(3):265–269.
13. Olson KR, Durwood L, DeMeules M, McLaughlin KA. Mental Health of Transgender Children Who Are Supported in Their Identities. *Pediatrics.* 2016;137(3):e20153223.
14. Bridges JG, Lefevor GT, Rosik RLSH. Identity Affirmation and Mental Health Among Sexual Minorities: A Raised-Mormon Sample. *Journal of GLBT Family Studies.* 2020;16(3):293–311.
15. Baams L, Grossman AH, Russell ST. Minority Stress and Mechanisms of Risk for Depression and Suicidal Ideation Among Lesbian, Gay, and Bisexual Youth. *Developmental Psychology,* 2015;51(5):688–696.
16. Eder D, Evans CC, Parker S. *School Talk: Gender and Adolescent Culture.* New Brunswick, NJ: Rutgers University Press; 1995.
17. Gallagher R. Uncovering Schools' Strategies to Support LGBTQ+ Kids' Mental Health in Divided Places. Paper presented at the Annual Meetings of the American Sociological Association; August 17–21, 2023; Philadelphia, PA.

18. Pope D, Brown M, Miles S. *Overloaded and Underprepared: Strategies for Stronger Schools and Healthy, Successful Kids*. San Francisco: Jossey-Bass; 2015.

19. Goffman E. *Stigma: Notes on the Management of Spoiled Identity*. Englewood Cliffs, NJ: Prentice-Hall, Inc.; 1963.

20. Pescosolido BA, Perry BL, Krendl AC. Empowering the Next Generation to End Stigma by Starting the Conversation: Bring Change to Mind and the College Toolbox Project. *Journal of the American Academy of Child & Adolescent Psychiatry*. 2020;59(4):519–530. doi: 10.1016/j.jaac.2019.06.1016.

21. Abrutyn S, Mueller AS. Are Suicidal Behaviors Contagious? Using Longitudinal Data to Examine Suicide Suggestion. *American Sociological Review*. 2014; 79(2):211–227.

22. American Foundation for Suicide Prevention. *After a Suicide: A Toolkit for Schools*, 2nd ed. Waltham, MA: Education Development Center; 2018. Retrieved 6/24/22. https://afsp.org/after-a-suicide-a-toolkit-for-schools.

23. Erbacher TA, Singer JB, Poland S. *Suicide in Schools: A Practitioner's Guide to Multi-Level Prevention, Assessment, Intervention, and Postvention*. New York: Routledge; 2014.

24. American Foundation for Suicide Prevention. State Laws: Suicide Prevention in Schools (K-12). Retrieved 4/26/22. 2020. https://www.datocms-assets.com/12810/1602535612-k-1602535612-schools-issue-brief-1602535610-1602535612-1602535620.pdf.

25. American Foundation for Suicide Prevention. Bring Suicide Prevention to Your School. 2022. Retrieved 12/20/22. https://afsp.org/bring-suicide-prevention-to-your-school.

26. Suicide Prevention Resource Center. After a Suicide: Recommendations for Religious Services and Other Public Memorial Observances. 2004. Retrieved 12/20/22.https://www.sprc.org/resources-programs/after-suicide-recommendations-religious-services-and-other-public-memorial.

27. O'Connor R. *When It Is Darkest: Why People Die by Suicide and What We Can Do to Prevent It*. New York: Random House; 2021.

28. Krysinska K, Jahn DR, Spencer-Thomas S, Andriessen K. The Roles of Religion and Spirituality in Suicide Bereavement and Postvention. *Postvention in Action: The International Handbook of Suicide Bereavement Support*. 2017;5:186–196.

29. Wyman PA, Pickering TA, Pisani AR, et al. Peer-Adult Network Structure and Suicide Attempts in 38 High Schools: Implications for Network-Informed Suicide Prevention. *Journal of Child Psychology and Psychiatry*. 2019;60(10):1065–1075. doi: 1010.1111/jcpp.13102.

30. Allen J, Hopper K, Wexler L, Kral M, Rasmus S, Nystad K. Mapping Resilience Pathways of Indigenous Youth in Five Circumpolar Communities. *Transcultural Psychiatry*. 2014;51(4):601–631.

31. Haenschen K, Tedesco JC. Framing the Youth-Led Movement for Gun Violence Prevention: How News Coverage Impacts Efficacy in Generation Z, Millennials, and Gen X. *The International Journal of Press/Politics*. 2020;25(4):653–675.

32. Leachman M, Masterson K, Figueroa E. A Punishing Decade for School Funding. Center on Budget and Policy Priorities; 2017. Retrieved 9/20/20. https://www.cbpp.org/research/state-budget-and-tax/a-punishing-decade-for-school-funding.

33. Blake MK. Other Duties as Assigned: The Ambiguous Role of the High School Counselor. *Sociology of Education*. 2020;93(4):315–330. doi: 10.1177/0038040720932563.
34. Brown B. Understanding and Assessing School Police Officers: A Conceptual and Methodological Comment. *Journal of Criminal Justice*. 2006;34(6):591–604.
35. Yip PSF, Caine E, Yousuf S, Chang S-S, Wu KC-C, Chen Y-Y. Means Restriction for Suicide Prevention. *The Lancet*. 2012;379(9834):2393–2399.
36. Pirkis J, Spittal MJ, Cox G, Robinson J, Cheung YTD, Studdert D. The Effectiveness of Structural Interventions at Suicide Hotspots: A Meta-Analysis. *International Journal of Epidemiology*. 2013;42(2):541–548.
37. Pirkis J, L, Too S, Spittal MJ, Krysinska K, Robinson J, Cheung YTD. Interventions to Reduce Suicides at Suicide Hotspots: A Systematic Review and Meta-Analysis. *The Lancet Psychiatry*. 2015;2(1):994–1001.
38. Kwong E, Chatterjee R, Grayson G, Lu T. How to Reach Out When Someone You Know May Be At Risk of Suicide. *Short Wave*. NPR; 2021. Retrieved 5/8/2022. https://www.npr.org/2021/04/02/983823424/how-to-reach-out-when-someone-you-know-may-be-at-risk-of-suicide.
39. Freedenthal S. *Loving Someone with Suicidal Thoughts: What Family, Friends, and Partners Can Say and Do*. Oakland, CA: New Harbinger Publications; 2023.

RESEARCH METHODOLOGY

In fall of 2013, Anna received a message on an online discussion board from a fellow scientist asking whether she did research on suicide contagion in adolescence. The person wanted help understanding what was going on in their hometown—Poplar Grove—which had been repeatedly rocked by youth suicide clusters. This message arrived at the same time that we were considering a shift toward qualitative methods, since we were unable to find data sets with the survey items we felt we needed to help us further understand how suicide contagion worked. We were no longer satisfied with documenting that suicide contagion was "real" using causal modeling strategies and longitudinal, nationally representative survey data—we wanted to understand how it worked so that we could identify strategies to disrupt it. So we took a chance and agreed first to a phone call with a community mental health leader, then to an in-person visit with a group of concerned Poplar Grovians who were working to prevent suicide in their cherished community.

While community leaders initiated this project—they chose us as it were, we were interested in the community because of the significant number of youth suicides, including youth suicide clusters, that the community said they had endured for years. Our initial goal was to understand how individuals cope with losing someone they care about to suicide or with having someone they care about attempt suicide. We reasoned that selecting our sample on exposure to suicide might help us understand what generated risk and resilience in the aftermath of this experience.

For the sake of gaining trust and being granted access, it turned out to be quite critical that we were invited into Poplar Grove. One of the most asked questions during our fieldwork was "Why us?" And it helped greatly that we could say, your community leaders invited us here to help identify new ways to prevent suicide and understand youth's psychological pain. No one wanted to think that their local reputation as a place with a "suicide problem" had reached us in our out-of-state homes.

A.1 OUR SCIENTIFIC PROCESS

Being scientifically rigorous in our research was important to us. If we want to suggest ways to intervene in Poplar Grove and other communities with similar problems, we needed to be certain—or as certain as is ever possible—that what we were finding was not based solely on our own perceptions and that our conclusions were robust. We couldn't just describe what was happening in Poplar Grove; we really had to build theoretical models of how suicide clusters form and persist and how the social environment places youth at risk of suicide. The way we thought about scientific rigor was that if another research team (with reasonably similar grounding in the literature and research methods) arrived, they would see the same patterns and draw the same conclusions that we did, even if, of course, they would put their own spin on it.

A.2 TEAM ETHNOGRAPHY

Our epistemological approach was guided by team ethnographic approaches[1] and abductive analysis.[2] Team ethnography is a methodology that helps limit one critique of qualitative methods—that findings are too dependent on the eye of the observer. While we do not believe that ethnographies that are not team ethnographies are invalid, or that they are limited in their ability to inform science (we believe quite the opposite), we did appreciate having multiple observers and analysts. We feel this enriched our ability to understand Poplar Grove, particularly when combined with an abductive analytic approach.

A.3 ABDUCTIVE ANALYSIS

Abduction is an analytic approach that encourages scientists to focus on surprising research evidence—evidence that does not fit our existing theories—and then to leverage those surprising cases to generate new hypotheses that—pending evidence—can advance our theoretical understanding of our social worlds. Or in our case, of how suicide clusters form and persist and how social forces shape suicide risk in adolescence. This means that we went into the field acknowledging that we had substantial knowledge of existing sociological theories of suicide, of social contagion processes (generally, and of the social contagion of suicide specifically), as well as theories of suicide bereavement and healing, and that this knowledge shaped what we anticipated to find. It also shaped our early hypotheses.

A.3.1 Our Theoretical Orientations

It is worth taking a moment to take stock of our knowledge bases as they shaped our early assumptions about what we would find in Poplar Grove. Prior to fieldwork, we had already collaborated for two years on suicide research, all of which was either quantitative or theoretical in nature. We were well aware of each other's favorite theoretical orientations and methodological trainings. While Seth is a general theorist, he is partial to social psychology,[i] the sociology of emotions, and most of his past work has focused on linking the macro-level social world (think: the entirety of society) to individuals' daily lives (interactions, identities, etc.) Seth was also trained in historical and archival research methods. Anna, on the other hand, largely draws on theories from sociology of education, children/youth (adolescent development) and medical sociology in her research to understand youth's lives in context. She is also partial to seeing the world through social network and social psychological lenses and has spent much of her career focused on how the meso-level social world (think: neighborhoods, schools) matters to individuals' life chances. Methodologically, Anna is highly trained in quantitative methods and has a keen interest in causal inference. While we both had some limited training in qualitative methods, we recognized the need to deepen that training prior to designing this study.

To prepare for fieldwork, we dove deep into qualitative methodology (Anna audited Prof. Zandria Robinson's course on qualitative methods at the University of Memphis). We also took care to review literatures that we were weak in, reading and discussing psychological, public health, and epidemiological theories of suicide and suicide clusters in particular. As fieldwork progressed, and we realized that Poplar Grove's local culture was massively important, we submersed ourselves in the sociology of culture. Later, we also reviewed the anthropology of suicide, thanks to guidance from Anna's colleague, medical anthropologist Eugene Raikhel. The anthropology of suicide is much stronger on the role of culture in suicide than the sociology of suicide (at least at the time!). Knitting these theories together helped us formulate preliminary hypotheses of why a community like Poplar Grove may experience recurring suicides and how suicide contagion operates. We used all of this reading to be careful about our assumptions regarding what causes suicide and what is known about suicide. It was fun (yes, we are nerds). We did all of this because abduction explicitly encourages the active pursuit of confirming and disconfirming evidence. To do that, you have to know a lot about what is already known, what there is to confirm or disconfirm.

A.3.2 Why Do We Study Suicide?

We get asked this question a lot, and since lived experience matters to the production of science, it is a reasonable if potentially sensitive question. Neither of us has ever been suicidal or has lost someone we were extremely close to suicide, though Anna has been highly impacted by the multiple people close to her who have attempted suicide or who have experienced suicidal crises, and she has lost students she didn't know well to suicide. Because these are not her stories to share, that's all the detail we will give here. However, even though Anna has some lived experience as an impacted friend or family member, this was not consciously in her mind when she chose suicide as a topic of study. But it has contributed to her enduring interest in the topic and in suicide prevention.

In truth, the story of our introduction to suicide research is the story of two assistant professors just starting out at the University of Memphis. We thought collaborating could be fun and could help us get tenure. Seth had some questions from great works of theory that he wanted to test empirically. He proposed we study either Émile Durkheim's *Suicide* or Erving Goffman's *Stigma*. Anna, empiricist that she is, dug into her data set to see what was feasible. No point if there isn't data! After doing a few literature reviews and reading quite a few codebooks from nationally representative data sets, she found a puzzle worth digging into: Is suicide socially contagious in adolescence? Our first paper was born.[3] In the process of doing this research, we realized how few sociologists were contributing to anything in suicidology or suicide prevention. And yet social contexts and social relationships were clearly critical to suicide risk and prevention. Suicide also seemed like a really interesting case to improve theories of social contagion, since exposure to suicide was such an intense and memorable experience, potentially allowing us to unpack things like exposure to emotions, behaviors, meanings of behaviors, and postexposure meaning-making. We felt that a broader, more comprehensive sociology of suicide was needed and could be useful for sociology and beyond.

A.3.3 Making Space to Question Our Assumptions

We began fieldwork with focus groups involving parents, youth, and mental health workers, in part to help us check our assumptions or biases about what life was like in this community. We wanted a broad, diverse view of life in Poplar Grove before designing additional study protocols. Our early questions were very open. What was it like to be a parent in Poplar Grove? What was it like to grow up there? What did they believe caused the mental health struggles and even suicide that kids were experiencing? Was suicide even a problem? This last question was not one we took lightly. We did not assume that just because some community leaders told us suicide was a problem that it actually was. Thus, another of our early tasks was to construct a comprehensive list of all the suicide deaths in the community, double-check and confirm the reports, and then use (the limited but publicly available) data from the local public health department on local suicide rates. Unfortunately, the local coroner/ medical examiner was not easily accessible, since they were located in a major city far away and had many barriers to accessing their information (particularly on our extremely limited budget). Ultimately, we were able to confirm that Poplar Grove has a disproportionate rate of youth suicide, including repeating suicide clusters—a determination also shared by professionals working on suicide prevention in the county's department of public health. A healthy skepticism and a determination to triangulate facts make for more rigorous scientific research. After getting to know the community through focus groups, we proceeded to our more intensive interviews.

A.3.4 The Surprising Finding

As we mentioned, abduction as a method encourages scientists to look for surprising findings, as those are the places with opportunities to advance our understanding of how things work and why people do what they do. The surprising finding that proved pivotal to our project appeared in our earliest focus groups. Past research—from Durkheim's writings in the 19th century to current public health studies—strongly suggests that high rates of suicide are more likely to occur in places that *lack* social connectedness. So we expected to find a really disconnected community in Poplar Grove, devoid of a strong collective identity and lacking in social support. We were extremely surprised when we got there. As we demonstrated in Chapter 1, that was just not the case. And we both independently recognized this surprising finding in our early fieldwork. Indeed, even the people who had tough experiences with the intense connectedness were quite clear that they loved the community and felt an abundance of social support and joy in their neighbors and Poplar Grove, as a place. And this contradiction held true from our first day of fieldwork through our last. What on earth was going on then? From a Durkheimian standpoint, and from a suicidology/suicide prevention standpoint, this was quite unexpected.

From a social networks standpoint, this was slightly less unexpected. There is some limited research on the perils of high degrees of social connectedness. For example, research by prominent sociologists Alejandro Portes[4,5] and James Coleman[6] anticipates some of what we found in Poplar Grove: that highly connected communities can have downsides, that they can foster the exclusion of outsiders and increase demands and expectations on insiders. And of course, social psychological research cautions that not fitting in is a fundamentally painful experience.[7] Still, these insights had not made their way into research on youth suicide, and they had not been unpacked so that we could understand how connectedness could go awry and generate unexpectedly high rates of suicide in a community. So we reoriented ourselves to this new research question and set to work.

A.3.5 The Value of Comparison Cases

In addition to being oriented toward surprising findings, abduction (and sociology more generally) also values comparison cases. Abduction cautions us to pay as much attention to them as to the dominant themes in our data. So we began trying to understand how and why they were different, and what they could teach us about life in Poplar Grove. It turns out a lot. In addition to comparing cases within Poplar Grove (e.g., the cultural rebels vs. the majority of youth), we would have loved to have a demographically, culturally, and structurally similar community without a suicide problem to compare our Poplar Grove case with, but that simply was not feasible. It took us two years of data collection to really begin to understand the importance of the local culture, structures, and demographics of Poplar Grove, at which point we had massively spent down our meager funds. Also, how would we find such a case? And then how would we gain the same degree of access that we had in Poplar Grove by virtue of them inviting us in (rather than us asking to be let in)? As two early career assistant professors, with no grant funding at the time, we just couldn't manage it. Instead, we developed a reference group of individuals who had lost someone they cared about to suicide but did not reside in Poplar Grove. We still learned a lot from this group, and even published a paper on suicide contagion that did not make use of the Poplar Grove versus Outsiders distinction (indeed, this paper is quite popular with Poplar Grovians).[8] But we acknowledge the lack of a comparison community to be a limitation.

A.3.6 Using Interviews to Understand Motives and Culture

In addition to leveraging abduction and team ethnography, we were also thoughtful with our approach to using interviews as a methodology. While interviewing individuals to understand their experiences and the meanings they ascribe to them—as we do in this study—is a time-honored methodology in sociology and beyond, we are also aware that talk can be cheap, as the colloquialism goes, and that there are methodological concerns about overly relying on interviews.[9,10] These critiques are grounded in a well-established literature that reveals what people *say* they would do does not always match what they *actually do* when the moment comes. Similarly, how people explain their motives for particular behaviors may not actually reflect what *truly* motivated them in the moment. Finally, people often try to present themselves as honorable, good people—perhaps particularly in Poplar Grove, where people clearly have such strong beliefs about what is "good" and "honorable." This last factor is also called social desirability bias, and it captures the human desire to answer questions posed in a socially desirable way, to meet the anticipated expectations of the interviewer. This is perhaps particularly important when discussing difficult topics like mental health and suicide.

Luckily, there are strategies to limit the impact these biases have on interview data, strategies that we employed. For instance, we documented and paid attention to nonverbal cues like the use of metaphors, jokes, tears, and nervous fidgeting (as Allison Pugh[11] wisely instructs interviewers to do). We also paid attention to when an interlocutor's story seemed too rehearsed and compared it to prior versions of the same tale, which we sometimes had access to through our archival analysis. We paid attention to silences, pauses, and struggles to find words. All of this emotional viscera reveals a lot about how the respondent feels about their story.[12]

We also deployed some of these nonverbal cues ourselves to put our respondents at ease and make it easier to talk about difficult topics. Kids in particular were sometimes quite nervous to be sitting across from a professor (however young we looked, being in our early to mid-30s). We dressed down for our kid interviews (changing clothes midday if necessary). We also did things like kicked off our shoes, let them break rules (they drank in a no-food-or-drinks room! *Gasp!*), and if it felt like it would help, we cussed (it comes easily to Anna). When we first met Becca, she said she felt comfortable because Madison had told her "Anna's really cool. Like, we e-mail sometimes . . . and she changes her hair and says 'fuck' sometimes!" Becca went on to say that this description of an adult "definitely excited all of our friends." Despite our hair, dress, and language, the kids were quite clear that we were in the "adult" category (even while the adults assumed that at least Anna couldn't be a professor yet, she looked too young). But it did seem that we were able to skirt the adult authority role and be more like a much older sibling or an aunt who was much younger than their parents (and we would like to add—ahem—that we ARE much younger than their parents!!).

It also mattered that we were outsiders. We have no personal ties to Poplar Grove. People regularly commented that they could tell us things that they wouldn't want to tell a local. For that reason, even though we had opportunities, we never used local field researchers. People were way too wary of the gossip networks for an insider to work. Of course, we were in some ways insiders, too. We are both White, middle-class, highly educated professionals with successful careers and sufficient academic accolades that made us legible to Poplar Grove adults. Being similar to the majority of Poplar Grovians while also not being a community member likely helped us build trust and fit in.

We also took pains to communicate that we were not there to judge anyone and that any emotion was welcome in the interviews. Sometimes, when it felt appropriate or helpful, we validated our respondents' feelings, sharing with them that others felt the same or that how they felt was a noted response among individuals like them in the scientific literature (obviously only when this was true). These proved useful methodologically as they often helped put respondents at ease, particularly when it came to talking about emotions they felt embarrassed about. For example, when a respondent stumbled in an interview and upset herself by "being all over the map," Anna reassured her that the terrain she was heading toward was okay:

ANNA: I don't always share things like this, but I wanted to tell you that you're not the first person to express emotions like the one you're talking about [feeling toward your friend who died.]
INTERVIEWEE: Interesting.
ANNA: So that's sort of . . . I don't want you to feel like . . . You're not the only one, I think that, I would kind of like to hear more about that, yeah if you can share, it's interesting and not rare.
INTERVIEWEE: Well, that's somewhat validating because I somewhat felt like a jerk about that, and it's not really something that [I've ever talked about before]. I don't remember ever really talking about with my parents or my sister who was in her grade [about it].

Acknowledging, validating, and not judging how people feel is critical to all sociological interviewing, but it is particularly important for talking about tough topics. Perhaps part of Madison's strong embrace of Anna wasn't just her ability to swear with the best of them—it is that Anna took her pain really seriously the first time Madison shared it and connected her to a therapist, who she ended up sticking with for years.

When necessary, we also shared bits of our own personal experiences. One bereaved mother walked into the interview and immediately demanded Anna disclose her own personal experience with suicide loss. Anna disclosed that she had never lost anyone to suicide—that lived experience was not a central motivation for her research. The mother then immediately asked whether Anna had ever lost someone, whether she had ever grieved, and when Anna disclosed that she had, multiple times, the woman softened. At least until she tensed up and said, "It wasn't a pet was it?'" Anna explained that while she had also lost pets, she had been thinking of her beloved Aunt Brit and Grandpa Q. This was acceptable enough, and the interview proceeded after Anna double-checked that the woman felt comfortable.

We also made sure that we took care of our own emotional needs *outside* of interviews, though this did not mean *not* being emotionally present or emotionally expressive during interviews. It would *not* do to be cold in these interviews. We sometimes shared our respondents' emotions, and sometimes that was evident. We had a strong practice of self-care and debriefing with each other (and with our close friends/family). We also had playlists (thanks David Bowie and Queen!) that helped us channel our emotions and prepare for tough field days.

But despite how hard the interviews were, many of our respondents appreciated the experience and felt it was "worth it" or even "helpful." For example, when Seth asked Scott how it felt to talk about his classmate's suicide, which had been really sad for him at the time, Scott shared:

> I don't know because I feel like what we're doing right now [the interview] is good. We need to [pause] we need to do something and this [research] might help somehow . . . I just hope it's worth it. You understand? It's worth feeling bad about talking about it but if it means it'll help someone not lose a loved one. So, it's worth it. It's that idea

that the outcome that's good for the greatest numbers. So, if I have to feel bad for a little bit to help some people have a better life, it's worth it.

Others thanked us for listening, for giving them the opportunity to actually talk through what they had experienced, or joked about it being a really healing therapy session—how much money did they owe us?

The one thing that respondents asked of us in return was that we use their stories to help other people and to improve suicide prevention and postvention. "I hope you guys can do something," Chloe told us at the end of her interview, adding "I wish you guys luck." We did what we could to help individual Poplar Grovians at the end of all interviews by reserving time for respondents to ask us anything they wanted to about suicide and suicide prevention, and by providing a lot of information about local mental health resources (resources we were willing to help connect them to if they wanted). We also spoke with teens about other topics—like getting into college and how one pays for vet school. No topic was off the table, though mostly they asked us about suicide, careers in mental health (including what exactly we did, where we worked, our "job titles"), and whether everywhere in the United States was like Poplar Grove—with its pressure and suicide problem. But of course, these individual efforts are not enough, and we continue to do our best to make change in Poplar Grove and beyond through our research, pro bono consulting, and public speaking.

A.3.7 Our Abductive Process

It's rare that researchers peel back the curtain and let you peek into their analytic process. But in 2016, we had an opportunity to do just that at the annual meeting of the American Sociological Association in a session on abductive analysis organized by Professors Iddo Tavory and Stefan Timmermans. We share here because it allows you, the reader, to see an example of how team ethnography, abductive analysis, and emerging data all came together to generate a new theory of youth suicide (which we published as Mueller and Abrutyn[13] and also Abrutyn and Mueller[14-16]).

To show you how we collaborated, let's revisit Jim, a father who we met in earlier chapters (especially Chapters 1 and 4). Jim loves living in Poplar Grove. He finds it to be "a very tight-knit community . . . [where] you feel like there's a network, a safety net around you all the time." But for some reason, that safety net that Jim loved so much did not help Jim cope with the increasingly difficult mental health problems his son experienced. Recall that Jim felt very judged by his fellow Poplar Grovians. "I can't say [that people in the town are judging me], but . . . I feel that they're judging me. Yeah, 'I'm a bad parent.'" For Jim, this perception of judgment led him to feel embarrassed about what his family was going through. We both found the case of Jim to be fascinating—in part because he was so honest and vulnerable in the interview (which was done with Seth).

As Anna read the transcript of Jim's interview, she honed in on how Jim felt blamed for his son's problems, which was part of a larger pattern of parents being blamed for the suicide problem that she had noted in the community. This blame was communicated publicly, but also privately. Anna saw this blame as a form of a social sanction for violating the expectations for good kids and good families that the community held. She also noticed immediately that the dense community connectedness made this social sanction both easy to deploy and very powerful for individual community members, which resulted in the suppression of help-seeking. In Anna's explanation, her focus on how social networks (where social sanctions are key mechanisms for enforcement of social norms) and how the meso-level shape individual experiences is apparent.

Seth's interpretation of Jim's experience was compatible but emphasized different elements of Jim's story. Seth, drawing on his knowledge of sociology of emotions, immediately noticed that Jim was using words that indicate feelings of shame. Shame is often difficult to name explicitly, so we listen carefully for words like "embarrassment." Seth noticed that the community was generating negative emotional (shame) feedback loops that end up isolating parents and kids further. Parents feel shame about the mental health challenges their children are experiencing, and that shame is generated through conversations—through the questions people ask—that subtly communicate disappointment to parents. This shame causes parents to withdraw from the community when they need it the most. They keep their painful struggles quiet, which limits their ability to get help for their kids or access the social support that they likely need. Seth also saw the importance of the connectedness in the community. It made the community feel like one great big "feelings trap" for individuals. The consequence was that there were intense negative emotions resulting from even the prospect of failure. Where Anna emphasized the meso-level, Seth's explanation emphasized the micro-level, how subtle social interactions with peers in daily life impact how individuals understand and feel about their lives.

By integrating these diverse insights, we could formulate a new theory of youth suicide. Shame pushes us to link the meso-level to the micro-level. It helps us understand how the characteristics of the social environment—in this case, the high degree of social connectedness and the high degree of cultural homogeneity (recall Chapters 1 and 2)—have emotional consequences for individual community members, impacting their mental health. Blame reveals how the structure at the meso-level matters. Sanctions are powerful because of the cohesive, connected social networks. It also highlights that social connectedness is a meaningful characteristic of a social group, and not just something housed within an individual. The structure of social relations that surround a person matters in addition to how many friends a person has or how much social support they feel they can access.

Both shame and blame also help us understand how much cultural norms and beliefs matter. The highly connected social networks in Poplar Grove are conduits for cultural beliefs that narrowly define a "good" kid or a "good" family, and because of these cultural beliefs, the networks become conduits for shame and blame. If Poplar Grove had different cultural beliefs, the experience of mental health challenges, and the experience of connectedness, would quite likely be very different. We then used these insights to offer a new social-psychological Durkheimian theory of suicide that highlights how a high degree of social connectedness can facilitate su-icide for some, if not all, members of a community or social group. For all the details of this theory, check out Mueller and Abrutyn.[13]

So while we didn't set out to revamp Durkheim, making him more rel-evant to 21st-century social worlds and the suicide problems communities are facing today, our abductive approach led us to this innovation. Without abduction and team ethnography, and without being open to surprising findings, we may not have come to this place. This matters in part because this theory also has real implications for suicide prevention. It points to new places to intervene to make kids' lives better.

A.4 STUDY DESIGN AND DATA

All of our research methods were approved by our universities' Institutional Review Boards for human subjects research.

The interviews and focus groups we conducted with residents of Poplar Grove (N = 97) between 2013 and 2016 were our primary data source for this study. Most data were collected in person, during our repeating trips to the community, though some interviews were conducted on-line. Among these 97 individuals who participated in interviews were 11 pairs of children and parents. The breakdown of the group was 14 youth (ages 15–17), 20 young adults (ages 18–25), 40 parents, and 18 individuals that we group together under the term "mental health workers" (broadly construed). Mental health workers are defined as individuals who played some role in the mental health safety net as teachers, school counselors, mental health therapists or clinicians, doctors, nurses, pastors, suicide prevention activists, public health officials, and crisis responders. Some parents also fit in the mental health worker category. In these cases, we categorized them as parents versus mental health workers depending on what was the main thrust of their interview data. This varied based on their individual experiences. Taking this broad approach to our interviews helped us capture diverse perspectives on suicide in the community and triangulate insights from different perspectives.

As we briefly mentioned earlier, we wanted to have some ability to identify what was unique about the experience of suicide loss in Poplar Grove. As such, we conducted in-depth interviews following the same protocols we used in Poplar Grove with a reference group of interviewees who *lived outside of Poplar Grove*. This is what we call our reference group. Our reference group is comprised of individuals who have lost someone they cared about to suicide (N = 34), 20 of whom were young adults (ages 18–32). Unfortunately, in the reference group, we found it extremely difficult to recruit youth. In our experience, you must build up a lot of trust with parents before you can interview their children about suicide, which we were able to do in Poplar Grove because we were also involved in the community and developed a local reputation for being responsible, caring adults who could be trusted in this way. We were not able to do the same outside of Poplar Grove, though we tried. For that reason, our reference group includes no one under the age of 18.

Table A.1 provides descriptive statistics for both our Poplar Grove and reference group samples. Our reference group had older respondents, as we already mentioned, and included fewer White non-Hispanic individuals but more people who identified as female.

In addition to interviews and focus groups, we engaged in participant observation whenever possible. Our observational data were largely used to enrich our understanding of life in Poplar Grove. Because suicide is such a difficult topic to discuss, our best data really came from private interviews or focus groups with two best friends or parents. Still, participating in the American Foundation for Suicide Prevention's Out of Darkness Walks allowed us to experience the community grief firsthand. We also attended other suicide prevention events, meetings of the local Suicide Prevention Committee (a pseudonym for its real name), and explored the neighborhoods. We drove across the bridge that haunts the community as well.

Finally, we did extensive archival research and document analysis. Two families allowed us to include their children's personal journals. One is the 3,600-word journal written by Aria. The second are excerpts from Quinn's diary. We use both of these documents with the permission of

Table A.1 DESCRIPTIVE STATISTICS

Poplar Grove	Percent	N
Youth (Ages 15–17)	13.4	13
Young Adults (Ages 18–25)	20.4	20
Older Young Adults (Ages 26–32)	6.1	6
Parents	40.8	40
Mental Health Workers	18.4	18
Female	76.3	74
Non-Hispanic White	99.0	96
Subtotal N	97	
Reference Group		
Young Adults (Ages 18–25)	38.2	13
Older Young Adults (Ages 26–32)	20.6	7
Adults (33 and older)	41.2	14
Female	82.4	28
Non-Hispanic White	91.1	31
Subtotal N	34	
Total N	**131**	

the children's parents in a way that was approved by the parents. We also systematically collected communications from the school (e.g., principal's newsletters, student newspapers, notices to parents about a suicide death), articles about suicide in Poplar Grove that appeared in the local newspapers, public social media conversations about suicide or mental health, obituaries, and any other items we could find relevant to mental health, suicide, or even life in Poplar Grove. We used US Census data and Geographic Information Systems (GIS) software to map the homogeneity of the community during our fieldwork—to see in Chapter 1 precisely how homogeneous and how proximate to communities of color Poplar Grove was. We also researched school desegregation in the 20th century in Poplar Grove's state, reviewed segregation indices, and tracked school data for the county using data from the National Center for Education Statistics.

A.5 RECRUITMENT

While our interest was primarily in youth experiences in Poplar Grove, we felt that recruiting a broad array of Poplar Grovians who had been touched in some way by suicide loss and bereavement was important to paint a complete picture of how a youth ending their life in suicide impacts their friends, family, and community. We also wanted individuals to define "someone they care about" for themselves. We conducted focus groups (or small group interviews) so that we could get a general view of life in Poplar Grove and assess generally attitudes in Poplar Grove about mental health, help-seeking, and suicide.

We tried to be as flexible with interview respondents as possible. We asked respondents if they preferred to be interviewed by a man or a woman (by Anna or Seth). Most did not care, though if they knew one of us already they preferred to be interviewed by the person that they knew. Two men were quite explicit that they could *only* be interviewed by a woman—a man was a dealbreaker—so Anna interviewed them. Anna ended up interviewing more of our Poplar Grove respondents because she spent more time physically in the community than Seth (though both of us traveled there for fieldwork). Seth interviewed more of our reference group respondents.

We also allowed people to form their own focus groups (if they wanted), to be interviewed in pairs (moms and daughters, spouses, or best friends), or in one-on-one interviews. People generally had strong preferences— they either wanted the privacy of an individual interview or the comfort of a spouse or friend present.

Recruitment of our respondents was largely through community organizations, including a mental health counseling center, two religious organizations, and the government-sponsored Suicide Prevention Committee. We also set up tables with flyers at community events where we could informally discuss the research with attendees, posted flyers around the community, and relied on word of mouth. Because of the intense emotions surrounding suicide, we did not contact any respondents directly unless they had given explicit permission for us to do so via a third party.

A.6 DATA ANALYSIS

More practically, our abductive analytic process used the following procedures. All interviews and focus groups were digitally recorded and transcribed by professional transcribers. Transcripts were reviewed by the authors for accuracy and then analyzed for themes in NVivo 11 software. Themes were found through abductive reasoning, which emphasizes identifying "surprising findings" that emerge from the data.[2] We began analysis by both of us independently conducting detailed coding of the transcripts to ensure unexpected themes could emerge from the interviews and focus groups. From this detailed coding, we established our major themes and then progressed to "focused" coding.

At times, we grouped respondents into categories that were discussed throughout the chapters of this book—for example, we categorized youth and young adults as help-seekers or not, or as holding certain beliefs about suicide or not. We made sure to categorize every respondent independently, then compared the categorizations for consistency. We flagged rare discrepant cases and, after a brief discussion, reached agreement in every case. This research received human subjects approval from our universities' Institutional Review Boards.

A.7 SUPPORTING DISTRESSED INTERVIEWEES

Talking about suicide can be extremely difficult, particularly for bereaved individuals who may still be going through the process of grieving and healing. We brought to every interview a packet for respondents to take with them that included the *Handbook for Survivors of Suicide* published by the American Association of Suicidology,[ii] fact sheets about suicide loss and suicide prevention, and summaries of local resources. We also had a clinician in Poplar Grove who was willing to be on-call if we needed her. She was also willing to see any person who needed help regardless of their ability to pay. She donated this to her community and to our project, and it was a wonderful resource. We only made use of it once, but that one time, we think it made a difference. Youth who volunteered for interviews—with their parents' permission—were generally not actively suicidal, or they did not acknowledge active suicidality. Still, when we noted distress levels that were high or the presence of psychological pain, we went ahead and talked with youth seriously about accessing resources (and in one case, connected a teen to care). We did this with adults, too. Generally, our communicating our concern was received positively.

Since the time of our Poplar Grove fieldwork, we have developed more detailed and involved procedures for supporting distressed individuals. For researchers wanting to do interviews with potentially suicidal individuals, we recommend getting training in suicide prevention. Our preferred training is the two-day Applied Suicide Intervention Skills Training (ASIST) training by LivingWorks,[iii] but we also use and recommend the LivingWorks Start online training. We also recommend developing a safety plan protocol and completing training in evidence-based safety planning (to learn more, visit www.suicidesafetyplan.com). Our protocol now is to complete a safety plan with anyone who reports suicidal thoughts, whether they are actively suicidal or not. Some of these changes have to do with advances in research on suicide and suicide interventions.

A.8 ON PROTECTING PRIVACY

We had to make some difficult decisions around community and individual privacy to do this research in an ethical manner. To start, all names are pseudonyms. We have also sometimes changed details about a particular respondent while taking great pains to keep details consistent with the original so that the story does not change. We limit this practice as much as possible, but we do employ it. This is common practice in sociological research on sensitive subjects.[17]

We also have to take special care with people whose stories we include in this book but who died by suicide. Even though suicide was more common in Poplar Grove, it was still a rare event. If we placed a particular person who died by suicide clearly in time, it would be immediately obvious to community members who that person was, and then they could likely deduce who the interlocutor quoted was, violating their privacy. Families and close friends often shared deeply personal and often painful stories about the person they loved that died by suicide. It would not be appropriate for this private information to be aired publicly. As a result, we use two pseudonyms for some individuals and for all youth who have died by suicide. One pseudonym—what we call our "public pseudonym"—is used when we are placing people who died by suicide in time order or otherwise are discussing them in a way that makes them potentially identifiable to community members. The second pseudonym—what we call the "private pseudonym"—is used when we are not placing individuals in time order. When we place people in time order, we take extra care to protect people's privacy, generally by only sharing things they approved or that are publicly known (or both).

Our use of two pseudonyms admittedly limits our ability to reveal for the reader the depth of our data about any one youth who has died by suicide or any one event (e.g., a crisis response). It can make it seem like we spoke to fewer people who knew a particular teen than we actually did. It also inflates the number of suicides in Poplar Grove if you count by pseudonym. However, we feel strongly that these downsides are far outweighed by the need to protect individuals' identities and particularly the identities of youth.

A.9 ON GIVING BACK AND THE COMMUNITY'S REACTION

The community agreed to facilitate our research *if* we shared our research with them and gave them advice about suicide prevention. We have done our best to do this in two ways. First, during fieldwork, we offered the community pro bono consulting on any topic related to suicide prevention or postvention (we still offer this to them; there is no expiration date on this offer), and during fieldwork, they regularly consulted with us about random decisions they had to make. After one suicide, Anna was able to fly into the community (three weeks later) to answer parent questions about suicide prevention and suicide contagion alongside an expert clinical psychologist (we did not collect data that night, as that was just for the community). We still stay in touch and have managed to come back to Poplar Grove whenever invited (most recently in 2022, to share our non-Poplar Grove research with the community).

Second, we presented findings from this research to the community on multiple occasions. The first time was during the middle of fieldwork. We made this perhaps strange methodological choice (as we tipped them off to what we were finding before the study was done) because we wanted them to have information as soon as we were confident the information was robust, but also with the caveat that the information had not yet been fully peer reviewed (Mueller and Abrutyn[13] was at the time working its way through peer review). This meant that Poplar Grove was the first to know what we found. It also allowed us to get their take on our findings before the publication process, as a final reality check for us. At the conclusion of our fieldwork, we returned to Poplar Grove, several award-winning peer-reviewed publications giving us the strength to present our research to a gathering of over 200 parents, teens, school staff members, and concerned citizens. While the majority of locals reported to us that they saw the truth in our findings, though it was hard to hear, some parents very vocally took issue with the suggestion that parenting in Poplar Grove was anything less than perfect. "How could you tell us to not celebrate our children?!" one parent very emphatically asked of Anna. Anna replied, "I'm not asking you to not celebrate your children. I'm simply pointing out that celebrations don't have to be public to be meaningful and that there are consequences when we put successes out for public consumption. Kids then notice the things about them that you don't celebrate, things that could be perceived as publicly embarrassing." Some of this news was not easy to take. It felt counterintuitive.

In addition to sharing our research, we did provide suggestions to Poplar Grove about interventions that might prove useful, such as Challenge Success, a school-based intervention that helps shift academic cultures toward less pressure, less social comparison, and more privacy (grades don't have to be public!). Some community parents were beginning the push to implement Challenge Success; however, these efforts were derailed by the COVID-19 pandemic that began in 2020.

NOTES

i.   Social psychology is a core subfield of sociology that is distinct but overlapping with social psychology in psychology. Our core journal is *Social Psychology Quarterly* if you're curious to see more sociological social psychology.
ii. https://suicidology.org/wp-content/uploads/2019/07/SOS_handbook.pdf.
iii. https://www.livingworks.net/.

REFERENCES

1. Evans J, Huising R, Silbey SS. Accounting for Accounts: Crafting Ethnographic Validity Through Team Ethnography. In: Elsback KD, Kramer R, eds. *Handbook of Qualitative Organizational Research: Innovative Pathways and Methods.* New York: Routledge; 2016:143–155.
2. Timmermans S, Tavory I. Theory Construction in Qualitative Research: From Grounded Theory to Abductive Analysis. *Sociological Theory.* 2012;30(3):167–186.
3. Abrutyn S, Mueller AS. Are Suicidal Behaviors Contagious? Using Longitudinal Data to Examine Suicide Suggestion. *American Sociological Review.* 2014;79(2):211–227.
4. Portes A. Social Capital: Its Origins and Applications in Modern Sociology. *Annual Review of Sociology.* 1998;24(1):1–24.
5. Portes A. The Downsides of Social Capital. *PNAS.* 2014;111(52):18407–18408.
6. Coleman JS. Social Capital in the Creation of Human Capital. *American Journal of Sociology.* 1988;94:S95–S120.
7. Crosnoe R. *Fitting In, Standing Out: Navigating the Social Challenges of High School to Get an Education.* Cambridge, UK: Cambridge University Press; 2011.
8. Miklin S, Mueller AS, Abrutyn S, Ordoñez K. Suicide Exposure, Suicide Risk, and the Importance of Meaning Making. *Social Science and Medicine.* 2019;233:21–27.
9. Martin JL. Life's a Beach but You're an Ant, and Other Unwelcome News for the Sociology of Culture. *Poetics.* 2010;38:228–243.
10. Vaisey S. Motivation and Justification: A Dual Process Model of Culture in Action. *American Journal of Sociology.* 2009;114(6):1675–715.
11. Pugh AJ. What Good Are Interviews for Thinking About Culture? Demystifying Interpretive Analysis. *American Journal of Cultural Sociology.* 2013;1(1):42–68.
12. Small ML, Calarco JM. *Qualitative Literacy: A Guide to Evaluating Ethnographic and Interview Research.* University of California Press; 2022.

13. Mueller AS, Abrutyn S. Adolescents Under Pressure: A New Durkheimian Framework for Understanding Adolescent Suicide in a Cohesive Community. *American Sociological Review.* 2016;81(5):877–899.

14. Abrutyn S, Mueller AS. The Socioemotional Foundations of Suicide: A Micro-sociological View of Durkheim's Suicide. *Sociological Theory.* 2014;32(4):327–351.

15. Abrutyn S, Mueller AS. When Too Much Integration and Regulation Hurt: Re-envisioning Durkheim's Altruistic Suicide. *Society and Mental Health.* 2016;6(1):56–71.

16. Abrutyn S, Mueller AS. Towards a Cultural-Structural Theory of Suicide: Examining Excessive Regulation and its Discontents. *Sociological Theory.* 2018;36(1):48–66.

17. Hirsch JS, Khan S. *Sexual Citizens: A Landmark Study of Sex, Power, and Assault on Campus.* New York: Norton; 2020.

For the benefit of digital users, indexed terms that span two pages (e.g., 52–53) may, on occasion, appear on only one of those pages.

Tables and boxes are indicated by *t* and *b* following the page number